WHAT KILLED JANE AUSTEN?

and Other Medical Mysteries

WHAT KILLED
JANE
AUSTEN?

and Other
Medical
Mysteries

GEORGE BIRO
AND JIM LEAVESLEY

TEMPUS

This book is dedicated to our wives, Kitty Biro and Margaret Leavesley, who have been our constant supporters, our sternest critics and invariably a source of ideas.

First published by Harper Collins, Australia in 1998
This edition first published 2007

Tempus Publishing Limited
The Mill, Brimscombe Port,
Stroud, Gloucestershire, GL5 2QG
www.tempus-publishing.com

George Biro and James Leavesley 1998, 2007
Cover illustration by Louise Crowe

The right of George Biro and James Leavesley to be identified
as the Authors of this work has been asserted in accordance with the
Copyrights, Designs and Patents Act 1988.

British Library Cataloguing in Publication Data.
A catalogue record for this book is available from the British Library.

ISBN 978 0 7524 4310 2

Typesetting and origination by Tempus Publishing Limited
Printed and bound in Great Britain

Contents

About the Authors

George Biro was born in Budapest, Hungary, in 1938, to an Italian mother and a Hungarian father. The family migrated to Australia in 1947. With such a cosmopolitan background and being good at languages, he harboured thoughts of becoming a journalist. His parents actively discouraged such folderols and recommended he find a more secure and socially acceptable job. So he became a medical student in Sydney; whether this fulfilled the parental criteria is a moot point.

After graduation George joined a group practice in Manly, New South Wales, as a GP/anaesthetist. Later he worked in Ryde Hospital in Sydney. In 1990, having acquired what he saw as the insisted-upon security and social acceptability, he reverted to his first love of writing to become a freelance medical journalist. His articles have appeared in various medical publications. This is his second book.

Jim Leavesley was born in Blackpool, the holiday resort in northwest England. He had early fantasies of becoming a Lancashire county cricketer, but again parental reproval—coupled with the obvious fact he was not good enough at cricket—soon put an end to that nonsense.

He entered Liverpool University Medical School, graduating in 1954. He migrated to Perth, Western Australia, in 1957.

After having worked as a GP in the same medical practice for 33 years he retired to Margaret River, not to grow grapes but to pursue his lifelong ambition of studying and writing about medical history.

Between 1978 and 1986 he did a weekly medical talkback broadcast on local ABC radio, and from 1981 he has been a regular contributor to programs produced by the Science Unit of the ABC, mostly 'Ockham's Razor'. He lectures extensively on medical history and writes a fortnightly column called 'Historically Speaking' for *Australian Doctor*. In 1993 he was made a Member of the Order of Australia for 'services to medicine in general and medical history in particular'. This is his sixth book.

Preface

Most of these essays saw the light of day in the 'after hours' section of the medical newspapers *Australian Doctor* and *Medical Observer*. Others have been adapted from broadcasts written for and presented on ABC radio.

Those in the medical newspapers were aimed at giving light, even comic, relief and soothing balm to doctors once they had ploughed through and wrestled to the ground the daunting and largely indigestible fare of attempting to resolve complicated medical cases or unravel the latest medico-political chicanery or come to terms with more stories of litigation against their colleagues.

Medical history was always regarded as a soft option or indulgence in medical schools; it never featured in examinations. Nonetheless, we are all curious about our roots and the fate of our forebears, and from the interest the stories generated it became obvious that their recounting held a compelling, perhaps morbid, fascination.

With this in mind, it was felt the anecdotes would appeal to a wider audience. So with the help of some judicious editing to cut out the most gory bits, a selection of bizarre, whimsical and ghoulish essays as well as off-beat, quirky clinical facts have been brought together in this book.

1

Kings and Queens

Mary I of England and Philip II of Spain

Mary Tudor, Queen Mary I of England, or Bloody Mary, had staunch religious convictions which made her unpopular in various parts of the country. But what nobody knew at the time was that while on the one hand she displayed energetic piety, on the other hand she had an enervating and disheartening medical condition. If it had been treated successfully the course of English history would have been changed. Mind you, she would have had to wait for over 400 years to be properly investigated.

Mary was born in 1516, the eldest child of Henry VIII by his first wife, Catherine of Aragon. Her father treated her very cruelly as a child, used her in a game of political cat and mouse, and often expressed the wish in her hearing that she were dead. Not surprisingly, her health was always indifferent—although details are sketchy, as the royal archives from Windsor only date from the reign of George III (1760). It is known, however, that she suffered from bouts of fever (perhaps malaria), anorexia and depression. Even at her coronation in 1553 it was said she had fallen prey to melancholy to the point of illness.

At the time of her coronation she was unmarried. As queen, she became a glittering prize in the dynastic stakes of Europe.

In the end her second cousin Philip, later Philip II of Spain, emerged as the frontrunner. Philip's father—the Holy Roman Emperor Charles V and Charles I of Spain—negotiated the marriage (Philip's second).

True love had nothing to do with this match. Both Philip and Mary were devout Catholics and opponents of Protestant heresy, but above all, Charles needed English support against the French.

To marry Philip, Mary defied the hostility of her people. Historian Hendrik Van Loon wrote: 'Stout British hearts trembled at the prospect of the Spanish Inquisition establishing itself in their midst, and stout British fists were clenched in silent menace.'

Charles set down reams of instructions; Philip must be devout, never trust anyone, never show his emotions. Above all, beware the perils of the bedroom:

'When you are with your wife … be careful and do not overstrain yourself … because intercourse … often … prevents the siring of children and may even kill you.'

At the age of 16 he had married the Princess of Portugal, who died only days after giving birth to Don Carlos. This first son of Philip was physically and mentally deficient; Don Carlos was to die in prison under mysterious circumstances.

Mary and Philip were married in 1554, and the Venetian ambassador reported the bride to be of 'low stature, had large white eyes, was very thin with a red and white complexion, had reddish hair, a low and wide nose, no eyebrows and were her age not on the decline, she might be called handsome' (which leaves us to wonder what he would call ugly). Philip was 12 years younger than Mary.

Mary believed herself to be pregnant on two occasions. Four months after the nuptials her breasts swelled and discharged a fluid, and she had morning sickness. The following month she thought she felt movements. In April 1555 she withdrew from court in anticipation of a confinement on 9 May.

The doctors assembled and a woman of similar age to Mary and who had recently been delivered of triplets was brought to see the queen by way of good luck.

In a flush of premature enthusiasm Philip was misinformed by the Princess Dowager of Portugal that a son had been safely delivered on 7 May. At Hampton Court, scene of the lying-in, Dr Calagila thought delivery might happen any day. That was on 22 May, but he covered himself by adding it may be as long away as 6 June.

On the strength of this, letters of announcement were prepared to send to Heads of State in Europe. The date was left blank. They are now in the Public Records Office, London, still waiting to be completed and posted; for nothing happened.

On 26 June Philip was informed that the calculation could be out by two months. On 29 June movements were said to be confirmed and milk expressed. Still nothing.

On 29 August Philip could wait no longer and left for Spain. He did not return until March 1557, some 18 months later. By this time Mary was 40 years old and her indifferent health was not improved by worrying about her barrenness. Philip stayed for four months then left England for good.

In his report home, the Venetian ambassador wrote, among other snippets, that besides bouts of melancholy, Mary suffered from 'menstrual retention and suffocation of the matrix to which for many years she has been often subject'. Significantly, he also added that she was so short-sighted that, a book had to be held quite close to the face, and her voice was rough and loud like a man's.

In the autumn of 1557 Mary again thought she was pregnant. Alas, she waited in vain; she was not pregnant at all. So desperate was she for a child that there was a plot to pass off a substitute male baby as her own.

Mary took her childlessness as divine vengeance for the heresies still being practised in England. So she executed eminent Protestant clerics like Thomas Cranmer, John Hooper,

Nicholas Ridley and Hugh Latimer. During her brief reign, Mary had over 300 of her own subjects burnt alive.

She also pushed England into joining Spain against the French. When England lost Calais, Mary bore much of the blame.

She remained well, until May 1558 when intermittent fever set in. No child was forthcoming, and by October she became febrile, confused and lost her vision. On 17 November 1558 Mary died—deserted by her husband and hated by her own people—aged 42 years and nine months. She was buried in Henry VII's chapel, Westminster Abbey. Her half sister, Queen Elizabeth I, was later to be interred on top of her, and both are there still.

What did she have? Certainly two phantom pregnancies, and with the discharge from the nipple, what sounds like so-called 'prolactinaemia'. The hormone prolactin is produced in the pituitary gland, which is situated in the base of the brain. Normally prolactin is released into the bloodstream after childbirth and stimulates lactation while at the same time suppressing ovulation, thus stopping pregnancy occurring during breastfeeding. If there is a tumour (or prolactinoma) of the secreting cells, then an excess of the hormone is produced; this condition is called prolactinaemia, and is nothing to do with childbearing and can occur anytime, but the effect is as though the woman has just been delivered of a child, hence the breasts secrete and she is infertile.

Apart from prolactinaemia, with her stressful, lonely and deprived childhood there must have been a psychological overlay.

In 1994 a research team in Lisbon found that the unusual conditions of a prolactin-producing tumour and excessive secretion of the hormone prolactin for no known reason are more common in women reared without a father, or at least one who is violent and alcoholic. It is a strange connection, but Mary could fit it on the score of paternal deprivation.

But from what has been positively observed, she had lack of menses, no eyebrows, a dry skin, a hoarse voice and ever-diminishing vision. The conglomerate of signs and symptoms together with her mode of death would seem to indicate a pituitary disorder, probably a tumour (possibly a prolactinoma) in that small but important gland in the brain.

The status of prolactin in the scheme of things medical and its place in a successful pregnancy was not elucidated until the 1970s, so Mary never stood a chance as far as a successful pregnancy was concerned.

What we need is a peek at the skull, especially the bony cavity or fossa wherein lies the pituitary gland. If our theory is correct, this would still show the erosion of the bony walls from an expanding tumour, even though the pituitary itself has long since rotted away.

The tomb was opened about 100 years ago, but the attendant Dean of Westminster was no pathologist, so the type of conclusion we are after did not emerge. The Queen is the custodian of the Abbey and decides such things as who opens tombs. Her permission to settle our idle curiosity is unlikely.

We are left to speculate—if Mary had received treatment for her condition, perhaps she would have had an heir and Elizabeth I would not have ascended the English throne.

What about Philip?

'Workaholic' is what today's critics would label him. Hendrik van Loon just calls him 'obnoxious'. According to *The Larousse Encyclopedia of Modern History*, Philip was 'Lacking tact and intuition, he ruled his empire through a vast intelligence network and was a slave to paper-work.' Still other critics considered him dull.

But such dismissals do not do Philip justice; as historian J.H. Plumb writes:

> … a distorted picture of Philip has been created … Protestant historians … have portrayed him as a dedicated fanatic, sitting like a black spider in his bleak cell at the Escorial, working endlessly day and night to crush the Dutch, to reimpose Catholicism on England … For these ends he was prepared

to imprison his own children, to assassinate opponents, and to rack and torture all who thwarted him.

... but he was far more complex and much more human than the 'ogre' of Protestant historians would allow us to believe.

Indeed Philip enjoyed fishing and hunting, and appreciated gardens, buildings, music, and birds and other animals. He had the largest private library in the Western world, and also collected coins, medals, musical instruments, jewellery and paintings. He also received respect and even love from many of his Spanish subjects.

He was a devoutly religious man, leading a serious, purposeful life. As well as God, Philip had to contend with the figure of his father, forever watching over his shoulder.

1558, the year of Mary's death, was a watershed for both Spain and England. Charles's death from gout finally ended Philip's apprenticeship. The same year, Elizabeth I succeeded her half-sister, Mary Tudor, as England's ruler.

The English alliance was as short-lived as the marriage of Philip and Mary.

The rivalry of Catholic Spain under Philip II and Protestant England under Elizabeth I dominated European politics for the rest of the 16th century.

Protestantism for Philip II meant rebellion and chaos, while Catholicism meant unity and devotion.

Elizabeth always tried to avoid open conflict. According to the historian S.T. Bindoff, 'She would cheerfully have fought Spain to the last drop of French blood.'

The struggle ran for decades—a subtle, shifting game that Elizabeth played so well.

At times Philip worked to overthrow Elizabeth. But he also negotiated to marry her, and she led him on. While he lived in hope, he appeased her. So when he was not plotting against her, Philip the Catholic monarch protected

Elizabeth (an arch-heretic) from the Pope's plan to depose her by force!

But Elizabeth showed little gratitude. She kept supporting his rebellious Dutch Protestant subjects and encouraged Sir Francis Drake to plunder and destroy Spanish ships not only in the New World, but even in Spain itself.

Finally, in 1587, Elizabeth reluctantly executed her cousin, the Catholic Mary, Queen of Scots, who had been plotting to kill Elizabeth and seize the throne.

All this was too much for Philip. After 30 years of struggling with Elizabeth, he finally sent the 'Invincible Armada' against England. Its failure was a bitter blow to him.

According to J.H. Plumb:

> The problems that faced Philip were as great as his empire. He was constantly at war … The Turks were an unending menace … the Dutch and the English were officially or unofficially at war with him for decades Philip could never be sure whether the English pirates might not appear—burning, ravishing and robbing …

Apart from Spain itself, he ruled an empire of 50 million subjects. From Madrid, it took two weeks to send a letter to Milan or Brussels; two months to Mexico, and a year to the Philippines, which Spain was annexing.

Philip distrusted people, and did not like to delegate. No wonder that he dealt with up to 400 documents a day.

And his health? Philip's pallor and fair hair had always made him look sickly. His diet was neither healthy nor varied. There were only two meals a day, both offering the same choice: soup, white bread, chicken, partridge, pigeon, venison or other game, beef and fish (on Fridays). Fruit and vegetables were not popular.

For his constipation, Philip received turpentine, emetics and enemas. He reputedly had piles, asthma, gallstones and bouts of malaria (some have also said syphilis).

The gouty arthritis that had killed his father Charles also ravaged Philip. By his mid-thirties, he had his first acute attack; within a decade, the gout had become chronic.

As his health grew worse, so did his political fortunes. Marshall Dale believes that Philip saw his gout:

> ... as God's rebuke to a servant who was not properly diligent in the holy work of exterminating heretics and winning converts to the one true faith. His disease ... largely explains the unspeakable cruelties inflicted by a man who was not basically inhumane upon the hapless victims of the Spanish Inquisition.

Some 35 years after his first attack of gout, Philip's episodes gradually became more frequent and more severe.

By his late sixties, one arm was nearly useless; one knee was rigid, and he could only just hobble around. But no one ever heard him complain.

By the age of 70, he was nearly bedfast; he could neither dress nor toilet himself.

His surgeons bled him over and over. To drain his swollen knee, they reportedly inserted threads which produced open, weeping sores. Infection wasted his frail body.

Philip did not want to die in Madrid, but in the Escorial—the palace, church, monastery and school that he himself had built to honour God—about 40 kilometres away. To save him the agony of a jolting coach, litter-bearers carried him all the way.

From his couch in the Escorial, Philip could draw comfort from the sight of the altar.

Bedsores and ulcers now made it too painful to move him at all; the stench kept away most visitors.

While the sun rose on 13 September 1598, Philip II, King of Spain for 42 years, clutched his father's crucifix. As the children of his seminary began to sing Mass, he won final release from his sufferings.

(GB & JL)

Marie Antoinette and Louis XVI
of France – and sex

The year 1993 saw the 200th anniversary of the beheading of Louis XVI (21 January) and his Austrian wife, Marie
Antoinette (16 October). To compile an essay on the
medical history of beheading would be difficult, its swift final-
ity leaves no room for conjecture, but aspects of the royal
couple's earlier life together do provide us with a few fascinating
clinical morsels.

In 1768 Marie Antoinette became betrothed to Louis, then
Dauphin of France. She was 13 and he 14 years old. Marriage
could not take place until after her first menstrual period,
and as this did not manifest itself until February 1770, the
ceremony was delayed until May that year.

She was an attractive young woman, petite, blonde, and
amiable. He was gawky, overweight, uncouth, painfully self-
conscious, and described by the Austrian envoy as showing
'only limited intelligence. Nature seems to have refused him
everything'. His only accomplishments seem to have been an
ability to hunt stag and to make locks in his private forge.

Not a propitious beginning, but worse was to come.

The nuptial bed was blessed by the Archbishop of Rheims;
and King Louis XV, the groom's grandfather, gave Louis his
nightshirt. As the monarch was a well-known lecher whose
string of conquests had included Madame Pompadour and
Madame Du Barry, it may not have had much wear.

The couple retired, and, half dreading, half curious at what
was to come, Marie Antoinette waited. And waited. The bulky
form beside her lay still, asleep. Night after night the same ritual
was repeated. The chambermaids searched the dauphine's bedclothes in vain for the telltale signs of loss of virginity, and the
coy beginning soon became a matter of common gossip.

Spies from the Viennese court reported back that Louis was
'very much like a eunuch in his figure, and possibly a eunuch

in fact'. The royal doctors were consulted and made reassuring noises, considering he was not yet mature and that in time, together with the right food and exercise, all would be well.

To handle the royal genitals seems to have been outside the doctors' brief, for they missed the vital clue—the unfortunate bridegroom's phimosis. This is an inability to retract the fore-skin or prepuce; during an erection, constriction of the penis by its non-retractable skin sheath causes excruciating pain. The remedy is a fairly simple operation.

So, not having the gumption to seek help, the youth opted out of his marital duties altogether. Mind you, there was no anaesthetic then, and the thought of knives flashing so close to the crown jewels would have caught the breath of even the most insensitive lad. So a stalemate was produced by name and by nature.

To her credit, Marie Antoinette maintained her composure, at least outwardly. The two apparently discussed the problem, and surgery was agreed upon. But Louis decided to postpone things until his 16th birthday, 23 August 1770; and then, wham.

Louis' birthday came and went. The surgeon was not called and the shared virginity persisted.

There was similar vacillation when he became king in 1774. As the surgeon spread out the instruments, the terrified patient fainted (surely that would have been just the moment to act!).

After seven barren years, Marie Antoinette's eccentric brother, Joseph, decided to journey from Vienna and sort them out. For the first time here was someone who did not mince matters. After a heart-to-heart he wrote to his brother that Louis was able 'to have strong well conditioned erections', but not complete the act. 'He introduces the member, stays there without moving for perhaps two minutes, withdraws without ejaculating but still erect, and says good night.' Pain for Louis, disappointment for Marie Antoinette and frustration for both.

The forthright Joseph went on in his blunt way: 'This is incomprehensible because with all that he sometimes has nightly emissions, but once in place and going at it, never; he says plainly that he does it from a sense of duty but never from pleasure. They are two complete blunderers.' He wanted to whip Louis 'so that he would ejaculate out of sheer rage like a donkey'.

Joseph persuaded the dauphin to have the dreaded operation and advised his sister thereafter to entice her husband into bed in the afternoon when he still had energy; as later, after a meal, he would flag. Her brother then went off to reaffirm his faith in human nature by sampling the delights of the Parisian demimondes.

Now, with the prodding of his brother-in-law, the deed was done, and when all was healed the seven-year-old marriage was finally consummated.

At the end of August 1777 Antoinette wrote to her mother: 'more than eight days since my marriage was perfectly consummated; the proof has been repeated and yesterday even more completely than the first time.' Smiles all round. Eventually, she went on to have four children, but only one survived to adulthood.

But Marie Antoinette had other medical problems. When writing to her mother her whimsy was always to use the euphemism 'General Krottendorf' when referring to her periods, and from her correspondence it is apparent that she had no menses for the first four months after arriving in France. With the upheaval and subsequent sexual stresses that is not perhaps surprising.

But the reverse happened when Marie was incarcerated in her dank cell in the Conciergerie from 2 August 1793, when she suffered from menorrhagia, or excessively heavy periods. To add to her overall ignominy the queen, by now 37 years old and white haired, had to beg for linen rags from her attendant to help staunch the flow. The maid tore up her own chemises for the purpose.

On the day of her execution the queen asked the guard if she could change her stained petticoat in private. He refused, so she took it off in front of him, rolled it up and stuffed it into a chink in the cell wall. The cell today is as she left it, chill and austere; I am not so sure about the undergarment.

As she left to mount the tumbrel, the queen felt a need to go to the toilet. Her hands were unbound by Sanson, the executioner, and she relieved herself against the prison wall and before a clutch of bemused onlookers. Her humiliation was complete. It was sealed by her being trundled to the scaffold, where waited an inglorious end to a tragic and unfulfilled life.

(JL)

Did a mutant enzyme make George III mad?

History has not dealt kindly with King George III. At school we learnt that his decision to transport convicts led to British colonisation of Australia, and that he lost the American colonies and then his wits. But historian John Clarke has called him 'the only Hanoverian who could be called a genuinely decent and good man'.

George was 22 when he succeeded to the English throne in 1760. Twenty-eight years later, soon after turning 50, he wrote to his prime minister, William Pitt, saying that on 11 June he had suffered 'a pretty smart bilious attack' which forced him to bed.

At the end of June, Sir George Baker, President of the Royal College of Physicians, advised rest at Kew. The king also had a spell drinking the waters at Cheltenham in Gloucestershire.

But in July 1788, a month later, George suffered pain in the face and had persistent insomnia. In October, he had severe pain in his abdomen; Baker gave a purgative and opium, and reported that the king was in an uncharacteristic 'agitation of spirits'.

His condition worsened; more colic and constipation, muscular weakness, intractable, incessant talking, excitement, confusion, fits, failing eyesight and hearing.

According to J.H. Plumb

> He talked faster and faster and rarely slept. The Prince [of Wales, George's son] was sent for and the King tried to throttle him. George III's condition deteriorated rapidly and his death was expected. The Prince sat up waiting for it for two nights in succession, fully dressed ... The King did not die, but they had to put him in a strait-jacket, and no one thought that he would rule again.

The king knew he was ill. Just like other patients of his day, he suffered not only the disease but also the cures: emetics, purges, bleeding, blistering, cupping and leeching.

By November, George was reported to be 'under an intire alienation of mind' and considered to be mad. The King's disability became public knowledge. The Stock Exchange panicked.

Parliament pressed the royal physicians for a diagnosis, but they could not agree. At last the Chancellor and royal family called in over their heads Francis Willis, who was both a clergyman and a keeper of a madhouse.

Willis brought a strait-waistcoat, his son John and three keepers.

They controlled the king by intimidation, coercion and restraint. If George refused food or even threw off his bedclothes, Willis clapped him in a 'winding sheet', or tied him to what George bitterly called 'his coronation chair'.

The Countess of Harcourt, Lady of the Bedchamber to the Queen, wrote: 'The unhappy patient ... was no longer treated as a human being ... He was sometimes chained to a stake. He was frequently beaten and starved, and at best he was kept in subjection by menacing and violent language.'

The Willises minimised his 'excitement' by solitary confinement; not even his wife, Queen Charlotte, could visit without their approval.

They treated George's resistance to his treatments as part of his illness. In today's terms, they simply blamed the victim. But we must not judge them by our own standards; their approach was typical of madhouse-keepers of their day.

By January 1789, the need for a regency was obvious. But when the bill was with the House of Lords, the king started to improve.

When George went bathing at Weymouth, an enthusiastic band followed him into the sea to play 'God Save the King'.

He remained well for the next 12 years, but had further brief attacks in 1801 and 1804. Yet, in his first 72 years of life, all George's periods of mental incapacity hardly totalled six months when added together.

But in 1810, George was reported to have suffered 'a decided return of his former malady', and never regained his health again.

'His Majesty's adherence to certain erroneous notions with some degree of consistence partakes of the true character of Insanity,' noted Dr William Heberden the younger.

Parliament enacted the regency of the Prince of Wales (the future King George IV).

Marshall Dale has a poignant description of George's last years: 'Stone blind and stone deaf and, except for rare lucid intervals, wholly out of his senses, the poor old King wandered from room to room of his palace...'

What caused the king's recurrent episodes? Some historians said the stresses of monarchy overtaxed George's modest abilities and caused his breakdowns. Some said he had manic-depressive psychosis (now also called bipolar mood disorder).

But in the 1960s, two British psychiatrists, Ida Macalpine and Richard Hunter, claimed that George III had porphyria, a metabolic disease, in which patients show an excess of porphyrin in their blood and urine. Most forms of porphyria are inherited.

The two psychiatrists supported this diagnosis by newly unearthed medical evidence of the king's health, and an extensive review of George III's ancestors and descendants.

Macalpine and Hunter scanned 13 generations over 400 years for evidence of porphyria among the ancestors and descendants of George III, and found 'the purple thread of porphyria running through the royal houses from the Tudors to the Hanoverians, and from the Hanoverians to the present day'.

In all, Macalpine and Hunter diagnosed porphyria in 15 members of these three royal houses. These include Mary, Queen of Scots, her son James I of England (James VI of Scotland), Queen Anne, Caroline Matilda, Queen of Denmark (sister of George III), George III himself and four of his own 15 children (including the Prince of Wales, who became King George IV).

On the Prussian side, there was Frederic the Great and his father Frederick William I.

Coming to the 20th century, Macalpine and Hunter found four living descendants, analysis of whose urine and stools confirmed porphyria.

Dr Lindsay Hurst has extended the Macalpine hypothesis. He believes that royal porphyria can be traced even further back, to Henry VI of England (1421–71) and Charles VI of France (1368–1422).

But some experts reject Macalpine and Hunter's diagnosis of porphyria altogether. In a letter to the *British Medical Journal*, Dr Geoffrey Dean wrote: 'I shall end more firmly by promising to eat my hat … if the authors can produce convincing evidence that they are right.'

We can never be sure.

Whatever their cause, George III's attacks did have one benefit; John Clarke has said: 'The sympathy aroused by the royal malady opened people's minds and eyes to the whole field of

derangement and stirred the national conscience about the
the poor and mad.'

(GB)

Some royal operations

One of the more memorable deathbed lines in history is
when Caroline, the dying wife of George II, turned to him
and gasped: 'I want you to marry again,' to which he replied:
'Never. I'll never marry again. I'll just take mistresses.' Despite
his poorly timed insensitivity, he had the good grace to be
weeping at the time.

Caroline's troubles started on 9 November 1736 with
abdominal pain and vomiting. She was blistered, and given
Sir Walter Raleigh's Cordial and Duffy's Elixir, popular patent
medicines of the time. Enemas were returned without result.
Indeed, everything that could be done for a queen was done.
Short, that is, of actually examining her to try to find out what
was really wrong. If the attendant doctors could have brought
themselves to do this basic medical manoeuvre, all would have
been revealed.

After three days of useless treatment, a surgeon was called
and for the first time a hand was put on the abdomen. To his
horror an enormous strangulated hernia was there for all to
see and wonder at.

The surgeon elected to incise the mass. A thin trickle of
discoloured fluid escaped, but produced no relief.

Two more days passed, the wound edges began to mor-
tify and turn black, and the court despaired for the queen's
life. It was on this, the fifth day, that her husband uttered his
immortal words.

Two days later, the bowel burst, flooding the royal mattress
with excrement. Caroline, 55 years old and mother of eight, bore
the suffering with great fortitude and died on the tenth day.

George was as good as his word. He never did remarry, though he lived for another 24 years. All told he reigned for 33 years, was the last British king to appear on a battlefield (Dettingen in 1743), and was the patron of George Frederick Handel, who composed a variety of well-known pieces in his honour.

George II's greatgrandson, George IV, is well known to medical history for harbouring an enormous infected sebaceous cyst on the back of his head. It first appeared in 1820 and when the festering wen became too noisome for decent society, the foremost surgeon of the day, Astley Cooper, was called.

He took one look, refused to operate for fear of spreading the infection to the brain, and withdrew. It was one of the shortest consultations in regal history.

The king took it in good part, but a year later Cooper was summoned again, this time to see his majesty in the Pavilion at Brighton. He arrived by coach from London in the middle of the night to be told the monarch insisted that the offensive lesion be incised there and then. Treating a sebaceous cyst at 3 a.m. was not the eminent surgeon's idea of a night out, and he bravely refused the royal command.

The next day they returned together to more familiar ground in London. There Cooper dissected out one side, passed the scalpel to his assistant, who did the other, while the king sat quite still. Astley Cooper's reward was a baronetcy (it is uncertain whether honours were heaped on the second surgeon, despite his doing half the job).

In 1862 the 72 year old Leopold I of Belgium went to see his niece, Queen Victoria. While staying at Buckingham Palace he was seized with the torturing pain of bladder stone. The queen's surgeon, Sir Benjamin Brodie (later to have a special type of abscess named after him) told the visitor to go home and send for Europe's best lithotomist, or stone remover, Dr Jean Civiale of Paris.

Civiale came with his patent lithotrite to crush the offending item. He had two goes, failed to grasp the illusive calculus, but did succeed in inducing bleeding, pain and fever.

The well-favoured Dr Bernhard von Langenbeck was then summoned from Berlin. He applied the lithotrite four times. More haemorrhage and rigors, to say nothing of acute discomfort, but still no ping in the bucket.

In desperation a plea went out to Henry Thompson, a young 'stone crusher' who was making a name for himself in London. With the brashness of youth he had the offending calculus in his grasp first go. There was no bleeding or fever as the oxalic shards were 'pissed away', to use the contemporary vernacular.

Lack of infection puzzled him, but in ignorance of the bacterial cause of infection in these pre-Lister days, the reason was almost certainly due to the fact that the instruments used were brand new. Indeed Thompson was later to recall taking them out of their original wrapping paper in the royal bedroom. The lithotrites of the other surgeons glistened with the scarcely rinsed-away urine of a hundred previous sufferers.

Leopold gave the young man the right princely sum of £3,000. He was knighted by Victoria and became the toast of London.

In 1872 Napoleon III was living in exile in Chislehurst, London. He knew he had a bladder stone and that year it flared up. The by now Sir Henry Thompson was summoned. He crushed the stone under anaesthetic, but only got half away. The remainder became jammed in the passage between the bladder and the outside.

Another dash was undertaken. It was apparently successful, but urinary symptoms persisted. A third anaesthetic was deemed necessary, but just before the operation Napoleon collapsed and died. No huge hand-out or honours this time.

A post mortem showed the kidneys to be bags of pus and in the bladder there was still a fragment of stone.

To fail when treating royalty must cause the odd sleepless night as well as loss of face. Yet things are not as bad now as in the time of blind King John of Bohemia (1296–1346) who is said to have drowned all his surgeons in the Danube when they failed to restore his sight.

But other days, other mores. As for Sir Henry Thompson, he became very wealthy, was one of the first doctors in London to own a motor car, and collected porcelain, wrote novels, exhibited his paintings at the Royal Academy and generally basked in the sunlight of success.

(JL)

Opening the tombs

Gazing on the dead long after their demise seems to hold a macabre fascination. Look at the hype which surrounded the discovery of the tomb of Tutankhamen; Beethoven's body was dug up twice to try and help diagnose his deafness after his ossicles had been misplaced by the pathologist, who was, incredibly, called Wagner.

Mainly out of curiosity, one set of graves which have been extensively ransacked down the years have been those of English monarchs. Let's look at a few.

William the Conqueror died in Rouen, France, in 1087, ten days after being thrown from his horse. He was buried at the abbey he founded in Caen, northern France, in a stone coffin so small the body had to be bent double. On instructions from the Pope, the tomb was opened in 1522 and the body said to be found in a reasonable state of preservation. It was reinterred. In 1562, the abbey was pillaged by Calvinists, and the bones scattered, with the exception of one femur. This relic was preserved and reburied in 1642 under a monument, which in turn was demolished during riots in 1793. Despite heavy fighting in the area of Caen during the Second

World War, the femur's resting place was undamaged. However, it was opened in 1987, and a thigh bone was indeed found. It was reinterred.

William's son, William Rufus, was shot by an arrow by person or persons unknown while hunting in the New Forest. Tradition has it that his body was trundled on a charcoal-burner's cart to Winchester Cathedral for burial. The grave was opened in 1968, nearly 900 years on. Among the bones was an arrowhead.

Richard I (Richard the Lionheart) spent most of his time fighting abroad. His body was buried in 1199 at the feet of his father, Henry II, in Fontevrault, France. His heart went to Rouen Cathedral. In 1838 a small silver box, believed to contain the heart, was discovered in Rouen. When the box was opened, the contents may indeed have once been a heart, but by now were found to be 'reduced to the semblance of a reddish leaf', according to Brewer.

When Henry IV died in 1413 it was said his body and face were contracted by leprosy. But when viewed again in 1832, his face was in complete preservation and adorned by a full beard of deep russet colour. Henry's face certainly was not leprous.

Historians would love to get a look at Henry VIII to confirm or refute the syphilis legend. He lies in St George's Chapel, Windsor, but nobody has had the nerve to ask Queen Elizabeth II for permission. Idle curiosity is not perhaps a good enough reason to go fossicking about among her ancestors. However, when Queen Victoria gave permission to survey the tombs in Westminster Abbey, the burial place of James I of England (James VI of Scotland) was rediscovered. He died in 1625 and nestles in with Henry VII, who died in 1509.

Charles I was beheaded with a single stroke in 1649. His body was embalmed and placed on public display for a week. It was then taken to Windsor and placed next to Henry VIII (who had died in 1547) in a space which that king had left for his sixth wife, Catherine Parr. The snag was that she had remarried after Henry's death and so was beyond the pale as far as sharing eternity with her former husband was concerned, and so she is buried elsewhere.

Following his spectacular denouement, Charles lay undisturbed with Henry until 1813 when workmen preparing a tomb (seven years too early!) for George III accidentally broke into his grave. The Prince Regent was informed, and together with the royal physician, Sir Henry Halford, he rushed round to take a look.

A decayed wooded coffin was found inside a lead one. A small opening was made and the shroud torn away. The skin was dark but the musculature of the face remained and the famous 'Van Dyke' beard was intact. He was easily recognised from contemporary paintings.

The head, of course, was loose and when held up to view it was seen that the hair on the neck had been cropped. The neatly severed fourth cervical vertebra was smooth, even and awesome.

Charles was returned to his resting place, but when all had been resealed, the severed vertebra was found to have been left out. Halford kept it, had it mounted and used it as a saltcellar. It remained in the family until 1888 when it was returned to Queen Victoria. She had it put in a suitably engraved tiny casket and lowered through a small hole in the chapel floor onto the top of the coffin where it still is.

Oliver Cromwell died of natural causes in 1658 (probably malaria, then endemic in England) and was buried in Westminster Abbey. At the Restoration in 1660, his body was dug up and hung at Tyburn, the execution ground near the present day Marble Arch.

The next day his head was hacked off, the body, buried at the foot of the gallows and his head taken to Westminster Hall, where it was displayed on a spike until 1684. It then blew down in a gale and was retrieved by a guard, who smuggled it home. Eventually sold by this man's daughter, it passed through several hands until left in a Canon Wilkinson's will to Sidney Sussex College, Cambridge.

It was displayed from time to time and was last seen publicly in 1911 at the Royal Archaeological Institute. This irreverent gorping was then considered unseemly and after much debate it was buried by the college in 1960. To avoid student pranks this took place at a secret location.

Between the years 1683 and 1710, Queen Anne had 17 pregnancies. All but one were stillborn—even the survivor, William, died in 1700 at the age of 12—and child after child was lovingly enclosed in winding sheets and placed in the tomb of Mary Queen of Scots in Westminster Abbey.

The tragic Queen Mary had been buried at Peterborough in 1587, but in 1612 was reinterred at Henry VII's chapel at Westminster by her son, James I. Her fine sarcophagus became the repository of numerous fringe royals. When it was opened in 1867, besides Mary herself and that pitiful roll call of Anne's offspring, there were found her own natural son, John Darnley; her grandson, Henry; her grand-daughter, Elizabeth of Bohemia; her great grandson, Prince Rupert; Lady Arabella Stuart; and sundry illegitimate children of the libertine James II of England (VII of Scotland).

Is it in the interest of science or for mere curiosity that medical historians would so love to have one last peek in these tombs? As things are, the authorities think the latter. Pity!

(JL)

2

Eccentrics, Reformers and Pioneers

The bizarre affair of James Barry

For a woman to succeed in a man's world, she has to be twice as good as a man. Luckily, this is not too hard! (Anonymous)

About 1795, a daughter was born to the Barry family in London. For some reason, it was an aunt and uncle who raised her. The latter, a well-known painter, James Barry, believed in encouraging both males and females to achieve their potential. But this gem of an uncle died when the girl was only 11. She took her love of learning from him, and also his given name.

At 15, 'James' and the aunt moved to Edinburgh, where she passed herself off as a male to join the University Medical School. No way could she have done so as a female; that milestone was still over half a century away.

Though fellow-students teased her about her slight build and hairless chin, she kept her secret safe. Her only close friend wanted to teach James to box, but she learnt the rapier instead.

At 17, she completed a brilliant thesis on hernias. At the early age of 20, she gained her MD by defending this thesis against interrogation by the whole faculty, and by discussing two of Hippocrates' Aphorisms. Much of this, of course, was in Latin!

In 1813, she somehow avoided the usual physical examination, satisfied the Army Medical Board, and started on her lifetime career in military medicine.

Soon she distinguished herself at the Battle of Waterloo.

Next she coped well with a cholera epidemic at Cape Town. There she also saved a mother and child by performing a Caesarean delivery. Well before the time of antiseptics and anaesthetics, this was an exceptional outcome. Soon she rose to become private physician to the governor of Cape Town.

Wearing high-heeled boots and satin waistcoats with padded shoulders, James won the favour of many ladies. Since she excelled at duels, the men didn't dare rib her about her high voice or the little dog she always kept with her.

By 1821, as colonial medical inspector, James was able to raise the level of medical care. For example, she decreed that only physicians or apothecaries should prescribe drugs, saying: 'Pedlars and hawkers of drugs ... do more real injury ... than the most virulent diseases.' She also drafted the enlightened *Rules for the General Treatment of Lepers* and complained to the governor about floggings at the prison.

Naturally such a stirrer made enemies. Headstrong and quarrelsome, James herself often went to prison for breaches of discipline, but never for long.

In 1845, aged 50, she got the dreaded yellow fever. James forbade her colleagues from calling on her, and asked that if she did die, she should be buried fully dressed. But her assistant did visit while she was delirious and saw that James was no man. When James came to, she swore her assistant to secrecy.

After a year's sick leave she returned to duty. During the Crimean War, 400 of the 500 wounded in her hospital recovered; another exceptional result. At 62, as inspector general of all British Army Hospitals in Canada, she worked to improve the food, water and hygiene in her camps.

When she died at 71, they found on the bedpost the sheet she had worn to flatten her breasts. Her unsuspecting valet had served her for 40 years.

Had the army followed her request for instant burial in a sack, James would have taken her secret with her to the grave. But they called in a charwoman to lay out the body. She was furious: 'What do you mean by calling me to lay out a general, and the corpse is a woman's, and one who has borne a child?'

The army authorities continued the deception; both her death certificate and her tombstone show her as a male. But there were many red faces at the War Office when her obituary appeared in the *Manchester Guardian*:

> Officers … may remember … Dr Barry … enjoy[ed] a repu-
> tation for Considerable skill … in difficult operations. This
> gentleman had entered the army in 1813 … passed through the
> grades of assistant surgeon and surgeon in various regiments …
> Upon his death, [he] was discovered to be a woman.

Over 80 years later the *Journal of the Royal Army Medical Corps* gave her a fitting epitaph:

> Whoever was 'James Barry' she has the distinction of being
> first—the first woman doctor of the British Isles. Secondly—
> one who has … served her country in all climates with distinc-
> tion, and if she preferred to do so by the only way available in
> her lifetime, by assuming the trappings of the male sex, all the
> more credit to her courage and pertinacity.

If James Barry was the first known female medical graduate in the English-speaking world, albeit a status gained and
maintained in heavy and lifelong disguise, who were the
true believers who slugged it out with the medical establishment to gain the first legitimate toehold for women in the
medical profession?

Elizabeth Blackwell, an American graduate of British birth, is regarded as being the very first.

The Blackwells were a middle-class family from Bristol, England. Elizabeth's father, Samuel, a sugar-factory owner, was a religious man and held unfashionable ideas on equality in education and independence for both sons and daughters. She herself was born in 1821, the third of what were to be eight surviving children. When Elizabeth was 11 years old, financial disaster overtook her father, and the family migrated to New York. Samuel died a bankrupt when Elizabeth was 17, whereupon she and her sisters opened a school and paid off the debts.

Although there had never been a female medical graduate in America, she was determined to become a doctor, partly to fulfil her father's ambition, partly to right the wrong a friend had suffered—the friend had died from a uterine disorder as she would not seek advice from a (male) doctor—and partly to satisfy an urge in her feisty nature to do the impossible.

After 29 colleges had refused her application, Geneva College in New York State agreed to take her. The faculty had initially refused her application, but agreed to refer it to the student body, stipulating that any decision regarding admission must be unanimous. The students foresaw entertainment and notoriety, and voted 'yes'—with one exception, and he was sat upon until he changed his mind.

Miss Blackwell did the then usual two-year course, grad-uating as best student in 1849, and by so doing she seems to have set a pattern of excellence that women in medicine have found difficult to shake off since. Nonetheless, at her graduation ceremony she declined to walk in the academic procession 'because it would not be ladylike'. Her success inspired the English humorous journal *Punch* to publish some congratulatory verses to 'Doctrix Blackwell'.

Although she was well received, almost feted, in New York, it was more as a freak than as a serious medical doctor, and openings did not present themselves. Elizabeth went to the more liberated Paris, but found that she could only get a job as a midwife. At work she contracted an inflammation of the eyes, which was diagnosed as gonococcal ophthalmia. In June 1850 the affected eye was excised, leaving shattered any thoughts of her being a surgeon.

Dr Blackwell was welcomed in London. At St Bartholomew's Hospital she was able to work in every department *except* gynaecology!

On her return to America she was refused every post at every hospital to which she applied. She began to lecture on 'The Laws of Life', became known about town and steadily built up a large private practice, mainly of young and indigent women. Ultimately she opened a hospital staffed entirely by women.

In 1869 she moved permanently to England, and in the teeth of great opposition helped found the London School of Medicine for Women (later the Royal Free). For a short time Elizabeth Blackwell was its professor of gynaecology.

Dr Blackwell never married but did adopt a seven-year-old orphan, Kitty Barry (no relative to her enigmatic predecessor).

Elizabeth Blackwell continued to write on medical issues throughout her life, eventually dying in Hastings in 1910 aged 89. Kitty died in 1936.

The first female medical student in Australia was Dagmar Berne, who enrolled at Sydney University in 1885. There seems to have been no overt hostility from male staff or students and she completed the four-year course without incident. Then she blew her chance of becoming Australia's first registered female doctor by electing to transfer to Great Britain to pass out as a Licentiate of the College of Physicians of Glasgow and Edinburgh and Licentiate of the Society of Apothecaries of London. Dr Berne returned to Sydney in 1895, practised briefly and died of tuberculosis in 1900 aged 34.

Adelaide University enrolled Laura Fowler as its first woman medical student in 1886. She graduated in 1891, but did not register until March 1892, again thereby denying herself the unique honour of being number one on the register. Nonetheless, Dr Fowler had a long and eventful life, including missionary work in India and being held prisoner in Serbia in the First World War. She died in 1958.

At Melbourne University, no less than seven women enrolled as medical students in 1887. All eventually graduated, but the first two (in 1891) were Clara Stone and Margaret Whyte. They went on the register at once, thereby pipping Laura Fowler at the post and have their names writ large in the history of Australian medicine.

Today in Australia there are more female than male medical graduates.

(GB & JL)

Francis Galton, the man who walked north, south, east and west

He was a rough-cut genius, a pioneer who moved from one new field to the next, applying methods developed in one to problems in another, often without rigor, yet usually with striking effectiveness (Daniel J. Kevles)

The Art of Travel (1855) by Sir Francis Galton was full of handy tips. If you were a long way from home and feeling under the weather, just drop a charge of gunpowder into warm soapy water and glug it down.

Sore feet? Blisters? Just make a lather of soapsuds inside your socks, and break a raw egg into each boot to soften the leather. You want to keep your only set of clothes dry when it rains? Take them off and sit on them!

Galton (1822-1911) was an English eccentric, explorer, geographer, author, inventor, meteorologist, anthropologist and statistician. Some have called him the father of modern psychology.

Just before his fifth birthday, he boasted that he could read any English book, say all the Latin active verbs and recite 52 lines of Latin poetry.

He must have been an insufferable brat. An expert later calculated Galton's IQ at over 200 (but gave Galton's first cousin Charles Darwin only 135 and Copernicus only 110!).

He studied medicine at Birmingham University and King's College, London. As a medical student, he proposed that there should be an 'index of curative skill' to measure doctors' merit and to regulate their fee.

He did a statistical study of the efficacy of prayer. Findings: though churchgoers all over Britain prayed every Sunday for the lives of the royal family, the royals did not live longer than others.

Galton dropped medicine when his father's death gave him an independent income.

In 1850 he set off to explore Syria, Egypt and the Sudan; then vast areas of South West Africa.

Hearing that Hottentots were killing off missionaries, he demoralised their ferocious chief by wearing a pink hunting coat, riding into his doorway on a snorting ox and telling him to stop!

Back in London after covering 2,700 kilometres in two years, Galton became a Fellow of the Royal Society.

He was one of the first to discover that we each have a unique set of fingerprints that do not change with age. After Scotland Yard put Galton in charge of Criminal Investigation, his Fingerprints Branch successfully identified over 100 criminals in six months. Today we still use his system of arches, loops and whorls to classify prints.

He devised a method to decimalise British currency; a method which resembled the one finally adopted in 1971.

At home, he rigged up a signal that told everyone when the lavatory was engaged: 'It saves a futile climb upstairs and the occupant is not subjected to the embarrassment of having the door rattled.'

Galton often said: 'Whenever you can, count.' He saw measurement as the basis of science.

This passion for statistics enabled him to prepare weather charts more accurate than any before; he also discovered and named the anticyclone.

Galton wanted to compare the number of beautiful girls in British cities. First he invented a pocket counter; then he toured the cities pressing the button every time he saw a beauty. London had the highest beauty quotient, while Aberdeen was lowest.

But his life-interest was heredity. We can only speculate whether the infertility of his own marriage spurred this obsession.

His genetic work on peas closely resembled that of Gregor Mendel, though he didn't then know of Mendel.

Galton was the first to separate the effects of nature and nurture by studying both identical and non-identical twins.

In 1859, Charles Darwin's *The Origin of Species by Means of Natural Selection* spurred Galton to look for ways to improve the human race. The idea was not new. Plato's *Republic* idealised selective breeding. To prevent the human race from degenerating, Plato urged us to apply to humans the methods of breeders of dogs and birds.

In Galton's own work *Hereditary Genius* (1869), he concluded from a mountain of statistics that, given a fairly similar environment; most differences in ability are inherited: 'nature prevails enormously over nurture when the differences of nurture do not exceed what is commonly ... found among persons of the same rank of society and in the same country'.

Moreover, Galton believed in one general ability, rather than in specific talents or aptitudes.

When a historian argued that it was their specific specialised abilities that had made Caesar a great commander, Shakespeare a great poet and Newton a great scientist, Galton quoted Samuel Johnson:

> No, it is only that one man has more mind than another. He may direct it differently or prefer this study to that. Sir, the man who has vigour may walk to the North as well as to the South, to the East as well as to the West.

Galton argued for selective breeding between healthy people of ability. 'It would be quite practical to produce a highly gifted race of men [obviously women didn't get equal attention] by judicious marriages during several consecutive generations.'

He urged the state to run competitive exams for hereditary merit, applaud the winners at a public ceremony, celebrate their weddings at Westminster Abbey, and give them grants to encourage their breeding!

There was a downside as well. Galton advised 'stern compulsion ... to prevent the free propagation of the stock of those ... seriously afflicted by lunacy, feeble-mindedness, habitual criminality and pauperism.'

He coined the term *eugenics* (Greek for 'good breeding'). In 1907, he founded the Eugenics Education Society, which influenced birth control, abortion reform, sex education, marriage guidance, family allowances and taxation. But Galton did not want revolutionary change. He would have approved of genetic counselling, but he would have been appalled to see eugenic ideas used to defend the Holocaust.

Galton died in 1911, at the age of 88. His estate funded a Chair of Eugenics at University College, London.

(GB)

Marie Stopes, champion of contraception

Jeanie, Jeanie, full of hopes,
Read a book by Marie Stopes.
Now, to judge by her condition,
She must have read the wrong edition.
(Skipping chant, London 1924)

One of the books sent to Princess Elizabeth and Prince Philip as a wedding present in 1947 was *Married Love*. It was a gift of the author, Marie Stopes, who in a covering letter said: 'It seemed best to wait until you were married, and I now send it in the hope that you may be able to read it together.' It needs some gall to be so presumptuous, and Stopes had plenty of that.

It was hardly surprising that, as with the copies sent years before to Queen Mary (mother of seven) and the by then 10 years widowed Queen Alexandra (five children), the gift elicited no response. Yet since its appearance in 1918 the book has sold well over a million copies and been translated into 13 languages. In 1935 American academics voted it 16th out of the 25 most influential books of the previous 50 years. It was just behind Marx's *Das Kapital* and just ahead of Einstein's *Relativity*.

Dr Marie Stopes was a determined, single-minded, querulous and highly intelligent woman whose public behaviour became more eccentric as the years passed.

She was born in Surrey in 1880. She studied botany at University College, London, graduating with first-class honours, and then went on to Munich where she obtained her doctorate. Her speciality was palaeobotany, and she was later to write the definitive work on the constitution of coal. She never had any formal medical training.

As a young woman Marie had a number of suitors, but they were only entertained on a cerebral level; if passion did exist, it was confined to skittish and ebullient correspondence.

She did chase one man to Japan, but it came to naught. On the rebound she married a pallid and sensitive fellow-botanist, Ruggles Gates. That was 1911. When they were divorced five years later she was still a virgin.

But she had not completely wasted her time, for during the final arid couple of years she wrote what was to be her best-selling sexual treatise, *Married Love*. In the circumstances it would appear to have been something of a paradox, but maybe it helped set out her yearned-for ideal.

The book was published in March 1918. Three months later she married Humphrey Vernon Roe and finally was able to test theory against reality. The wedding was solemnised by the Bishop of Birmingham, who, in a madcap moment of abstraction, had himself asked for her hand a short time before.

The book was the first 'sex manual' in the English language and its mere 116 pages meant that lusty teenagers could easily hold and read it under the bedclothes. Alternatively, it could be folded within the covers of the Anglican prayerbook. At one London club it was in such demand that members were allowed to read it for only an hour at a time.

Today we wonder at its innocent, even puritanical, nature, but then it was dynamite. It spoke of 'stirring a chaste partner to physical love'. It blamed a wife's 'coldness' on the husband's 'want of art', and called for the 'profound mutual rousing of passion'. It contained contraceptive advice and extolled the liberation of women from the yoke of childbearing and male insensitivity. Its hitherto unknown free-thinking ethos was heady stuff and ensured the book's immediate success. It ran to six reprints in six months.

Dr Stopes became a national figure with a vast correspondence, much of which revealed the depth of sexual misery and prejudice within the population. Clergymen featured large among the letter writers. An Essex vicar wrote about his frigid wife: 'She is slow to rouse, once or twice a year … I am afraid I bore her … Single lust is a feeble squib; I want fireworks.'

One from Gosport: 'If I have touched my wife near the entrance she is much more "lively" … I feel dreadful having written so frankly.' Another from Newark: 'how best to arouse … my Wife always lies with her back to me, I make a "tender advance" … and the end of the poetry is "I do not like your breath on my face".'

A comi-tragedy unfurled, which was sometimes leavened by missives from the likes of the ubiquitous 'Disgusted'. One such with nine children angrily wrote: 'If God sends the babies, he will also send their breeches.'

Perhaps the most poignant was from a Yorkshireman who wrote about alternative methods of contraception. For him it amounted to 'rubbing "stuff" out of penis by hand of either self, wife or a middle aged widowed cook in absence of wife'. The mind boggles.

The medical profession was divided. Apart from obstetrics, sexual physiology was not taught at medical school; indeed there was precious little to teach. Knowledge of hormones was in its infancy, and all, including Stopes, thought the 'safe' period was in the middle of the month—we now know that this is, in fact, the most fertile period.

To the profession's amused contempt Stopes opened a birth-control clinic in 1921, mainly fitting cervical caps. It made a slow start but enough to outrage the Catholic Church, which intensified the scorn and vilification it had heaped upon her for the previous three years.

Though she had been denounced as immoral, Stopes held her hand. Then Dr Sutherland, a staunch Catholic, wrote that she was conducting 'a monstrous campaign of harmful methods' (cervical cap), and 'a class conspiracy against the poor'.

Although Sutherland's words were mild when compared with the usual abuse, she snapped and sued for libel. Sutherland won, but obtained a derisory £200 damages. Stopes appealed and the judgment was reversed. The Catholic Church was not to be denied, however, and appealed to the House of Lords inviting monetary contributions from 'right minded people'. Three of the five Law Lords were over 80 years of age, and Stopes lost 4-1. Sales of *Married Love* reached the half million mark.

Over the next 20 years Dr Stopes undertook numerous other legal battles with varying success. She also wrote two more big sellers, *Wise Parenthood* and *Radiant Motherhood* (both before her only child was born), but *Married Love* stands supreme.

She and her second husband became estranged after 10 troubled years of marriage. She treated her son, Harry, in a bizarre way, not allowing him to read until he was 10, forcing him to have only carrots in the morning, and dressing him in knitted frocks so as not to interfere with the growth of his genitals. In the end mother and son fell out and she cut him out of her will.

Although she was certain she would live to be 120, Marie Stopes died in 1958, aged 78. While regarded by many as paranoid and/or a deluded megalomaniac, it was the very nature of her overdrawn personality and unappeasable pugnacity which allowed the emotive subject of sex to be thrust into the full sunshine for the first time. It remains there today.

(JL)

Elizabeth Kenny, the bush nurse who took on the doctors

I was supposed to get married ... to justify my existence
(Elizabeth Kenny)

How can we explain this woman who was called both a fraud and a medical genius, a cheap quack and an unhappy martyr, a raging old tiger and a merciful angel?
(Victor Cohn)

Elizabeth Kenny was born in Warialda, New South Wales, in 1880. After several moves, the family settled on the Darling Downs in Queensland.

She planned to work as a missionary in India, but at 33, she became a volunteer nurse in a local maternity hospital. Next she was an unpaid visiting bush nurse in Queensland, by necessity often acting also as doctor and midwife.

In 1911, when Kenny was 31, she saw a feverish girl aged two, who was paralysed in one arm and both legs. By telegraph, Kenny consulted her friend Dr Aeneas McDonnell, who could only advise: 'Infantile paralysis (polio). No known treatment. Do the best you can … '

Kenny tried poultices without result, so she applied bits of blanket soaked in hot water. Soon she started moving the paralysed limbs and also encouraged the girl herself to try to move them. Moving limbs affected by polio was medical heresy, but Kenny did the same with five other children. Dr McDonnell was surprised to hear that all did well.

In 1915, she enlisted in the Australian Imperial Forces. From Nurse, she rose to Staff-Nurse, and later to Sister. While serving in France, she herself was wounded, and won a British War Medal.

After the war, Kenny returned to bush nursing. According to the accepted teaching of the day, since polio weakened affected muscles, these weak muscles needed splinting. Without splinting, people believed, the unaffected strong muscles would pull the weak ones out of place. Doctors 'knew' all this. With her usual total confidence, Elizabeth Kenny disagreed: 'No, I see only tight, shortened muscles in spasm—your splints and casts are illogical; throw them out.'

She invented and patented a stretcher that enabled people in shock to receive treatment while being transported.

In the polio epidemic of 1933, she used her royalties to open a free clinic in a Townsville backyard. There she treated patients disabled by polio. She replaced the conventional splints, braces and callipers with salt baths, foments, and exercises.

The following year the Queensland government appointed staff to work with Kenny to research unfantile paralysis. The 'Kenny Clinic' was the first nursing research clinic in Australia.

Her results impressed a few doctors, but most opposed her vigorously; one of the latter wrote: 'This quack must be exposed.' But Kenny clinics opened in Townsville, Cairns, Rockhampton, Toowoomba, Newcastle, Sydney and Melbourne.

One headline acclaimed her as 'A new Australian Florence Nightingale'.

Her public support grew and grew, and not only in Australia. Grateful parents of children she had helped paid her fare to England, where she cared for inpatients at Queen Mary's Hospital in Surrey.

In 1935, the Queensland Government appointed a Royal Commission of doctors to review the treatment of polio. After three years, they reported: 'The abandonment of immobilisation is a grievous error.' However, the report was never requested nor presented to Parliament.

The government nevertheless gave her a ward at the Brisbane Hospital. Here she could treat early cases of polio, who might respond better than older cases.

Kenny's few medical friends convinced the government to pay her fare to the United States. Many American doctors rejected her explanations, with some accusing her of using hypnosis. But she did gain the use of beds at the Minneapolis General Hospital, and the support of three orthopaedic doctors. One of these, Dr John Pohl, wrote:

> Before she came … you would have seen little kids lying stiff and rigid, crying with pain … We'd take children to the operating room straighten them out under anaesthetic, and put them in plaster casts. When they woke up, they screamed. The next day they still cried from the pain. That was the accepted and universal treatment … She said, 'That's all wrong.'

In 1941, the American Medical Association endorsed the Kenny treatment that the Queensland Royal Commission had rubbished five years earlier.

Doctors and physiotherapists from Greece, Russia, Turkey, Belgium, Germany, Sweden and China flocked to learn her methods at the Sister Kenny Institute in Minneapolis.

The *New York Sun* named her the world's 'Outstanding Woman of the Year'. In 1950, America awarded her Free Passage across its borders; an honour Elizabeth Kenny shared with French General La Fayette.

Many grateful people remembered that for over 20 years, she never took a penny for her work.

But Elizabeth Kenny herself and her teachings remained controversial. Her dogmatic belief in her own God-given gifts actually hindered her cause. She was merciless with anyone who dared to doubt her. Had she been gentler, could she have been more effective? Or would the critics have just ground her down?

She published two textbooks on her treatment of polio, as well as an autobiography and was awarded three honorary doctorates from leading American universities for her contribution to polio research. In 1951 she retired to Toowoomba, where she died a year later.

The *Sydney Morning Herald* mourned 'the loss of one of our great ones'.

The influential *British Medical Journal* said:

> The influence of Sister Kenny on the treatment of infantile paralysis has been exceedingly beneficial...in an empirical way she hit on much that was good in the treatment of poliomyelitis, and...wakened orthopaedic surgeons and physiotherapists the world over.

Sadly Elizabeth Kenny herself did not live to see this blessing by the medical establishment. The world has gradually accepted modifications of her teaching on the treatment of polio.

(GB)

Paul White, Jungle Doctor

Dr Paul White, the Jungle Doctor from Australia, earned for his work in the 1930s in Tanganyika, East Africa. There, despite his lifelong asthma, he was far more than a medical missionary: he was a surgeon, anaesthetist, pathologist, pharmacist, handyman and building supervisor.

Dr White learnt his first lessons in hygiene and public health as a small boy in Bowral:

> Before dawn, each Friday, a shadowy figure would come to our outhouse and play his key part in our pan-and-fly hygiene system. He was also our mayor, carrying off all his ceremonial duties spruce and shining in his robes of office.
>
> At a Christmas party, one of my mother's staidest friends asked me for a poem. I recited one our mayor had left us:
> 'Although the police keep order
> There's no more useful man
> Than the bloke who comes at sunrise
> And juggles with the pan.'
> To my amazement, they stopped me.

In 1921, his widowed mother and young Paul moved to Sydney. At Sydney Grammar School, he became a runner, cricketer and active Christian. He started his medical course in 1929, at the height of the Depression.

Paul gained a University Blue in 1931 and 1932.

> In my third year, I ran in the Intervarsity athletics. A Melbourne runner, Wellesley Hannah, beat me over the mile. Then I found that he was also a committed Christian. This friendship was to change both our lives.
>
> As medical students, we followed the desperate search for weapons against the great killers like pneumonia and meningitis. I felt especially bitter about meningitis which had killed my father.

By the time I graduated in 1935, I'd decided to work as a medical missionary in East Africa. First I spent one year at Royal North Shore Hospital, where our training included infectious diseases and obstetrics. For anaesthetics, we used the old ether with a rag and bottle.

As interns we earned eleven [shillings] and threepence a week and had every third weekend off.

In my spare time, I practised tracheotomy [emergency opening of the windpipe to bypass blockage] on an old piece of garden hose. Soon after, I had to do the real thing on a small boy who had severe diphtheria and couldn't breathe.

He met many challenges during his preparations:

Most of our equipment was borrowed: if we couldn't get it, we had to make it; if we couldn't make it, we had to go without. Mosquito nets were crucial, since mosquitoes transmit malaria, yellow fever, dengue and elephantiasis.

Among the things he learned: keeping a corrugated-iron roof cool, making a surgical retractor from two bent spoons, driving through mud or sand, and plugging a hole in a radiator or petrol tank.

In 1937 Dr White, with his wife Mary and son David, sailed to Dar-es-Salaam, the capital of Tanganyika (now Tanzania). Then to Dodoma and Mvumi.

Sechela the head nurse welcomed us with her story of a cobra emerging from its hole to watch her delivering twins.

Over 100 people came for my first outpatient session; some walked 50 kilometres. Relatives led the elderly who were blinded by cataracts. We had so few medicine bottles that people brought their own.

Those with malaria shivered in the scorching sun. Our only antimalarial was quinine, which we bought from the Tanganyika

Post Office for two shillings per 100 tablets.

Our operating room of granite, cement and corrugated iron cost 120 pounds. A burly African pedalling a jacked-up bike which charged a battery, gave most of our light. We built our anaesthetic machine from a pickle bottle, a car footpump, a football bladder, the Y-piece from a stethoscope, an eye-dropper glass and rubber tubing. It worked really well.

I removed many cataracts; trachoma I treated with surgery and zinc sulphate drops that cost threepence.

Twelve times a day, out two water carriers made their round trip of over three kilometers. Each carried 36 litres in petrol cans. Twice a week, the mailbag came, along the paths where lions and rhinoceros prowled.

The dry season lasted eight months and ended in October with torrential rain. Within minutes, a parched riverbed became a torrent. Within two days, grass would grow. We built water tanks to see us through the next dry, only to see them cracked by an earthquake. In one hour, we helplessly watched three months' water disappear.

Once sulphonamide drugs were discovered, we could fight the next epidemic of meningitis.

Our second child Rosemary was born in 1939. After my wife's illness forced us to return home, Wellesley Hannah came to Tanganyika to take over from me. He stayed 20 years.

Dr White's *Jungle Doctor* books numbered 54 and have appeared in over 100 languages. In 1977, he published an autobiography titled *Alias Jungle Doctor*. Later he was awarded the Order of Australia Medal (OAM) for services to religious welfare. Dr White died in 1992, at the age of 82.

(GB)

Bertram Wainer, abortion law reformer

I did not set out to be a reformer; I ... became involved with
a law which was inflicting human suffering (Bertram Wainer)

Melbourne, 1968. She was 21, and had already had a baby at
15. Now she was pregnant again. Terrified of telling her father,
she took an overdose and landed in a psychiatric hospital. Then
she threatened Dr Bertram Wainer that she would kill herself
if he didn't terminate her pregnancy.

Not only did he do the abortion, but he told the Press,
the Homicide Squad, the Chief Secretary and the Attorney-
General. Dr Wainer was relying on a 1969 judgment of Mr
Justice Menhennitt: 'A lawful abortion is one believed by the
doctor to be necessary to preserve the woman from serious
danger to her life or her mental health.'

Dr Wainer's challenge did not provoke any legal response,
but it marked his entry into the campaign that Australian
women were fighting for the right to legal abortions done
openly by capable doctors.

In the 1960s there were about 70,000 women having abortions in Australia each year; many abortions were performed
by unqualified abortionists.

Dr Wainer fought against strict abortion laws and their
narrow interpretation. He fought also against the police
corruption that he felt was a consequence of those laws. By proving the extent of police corruption feeding on undercover and
backyard abortionists, he forced society to face both issues.

His efforts helped to clean up the Victorian police force
and to bring about a more liberal interpretation of abortion
laws. (Nowadays, in most states of Australia, a woman can get
an abortion on demand, in the early stages of her pregnancy,
if her physical or mental health is in danger.)

Wainer's outspoken views brought him abuse, vilification,
threats and even attempts on his life. The Australian Medical

Association found him guilty of unprofessional conduct. Rumours said he was mad and had a criminal background. Criminals shot at him and tried to run him over. For years he lived in fear of his life.

What made a man fight at such personal cost for the right of Australian women to have safe and legal abortions?

His background gives us some clue. His father died soon after Bertram Wainer was born in Edinburgh in 1928. His stepfather was an illiterate alcoholic. Bertram's mother's sweet shop failed during the Depression, forcing the family to live in the slums of Glasgow.

The Second World War added more traumas. During the Blitz, young Bert and his mother were caught in an air raid away from home:

> ... bombs (were) exploding around us, ack–ack screaming ... fires devouring houses, incendiary bombs blazing ... then the relief of reaching an air-raid shelter. We were told: 'You can't come in here, this is a private air-raid shelter ... We have carpets and heaters and food. We can't let just anyone in.' The door slammed ...

Bert Wainer never forgot this experience.

He left school at 13 to help his mother, and was still under-age when he entered the army, where he served for the rest of the war. In 1949, the family migrated on free passages to Australia.

Supporting himself with a remarkable range of jobs, he somehow managed not only to matriculate but also to study medicine at Melbourne University. By the mid-1960s, he was a lieutenant-colonel in charge of a large military hospital.

After leaving the army in protest against the Vietnam war, Dr Wainer became a GP in St Kilda. In 1969, he went to the Press with evidence of backyard abortionists paying senior police large bribes for protection.

In June of the same year, radio station 2GB invited him to Sydney to debate abortion law reform. Before he left Melbourne, Dr Wainer told reporters that he planned to put before the New South Wales Chief Commissioner of Police (Norman Allan) evidence on abortion and police corruption in that state.

The threatening phone calls increased: 'If Wainer goes to Sydney, he will never come back alive.' The evening before the trip, a man offered to sell him protection in the shape of a shortened shotgun.

Dr Wainer and two trusted friends booked a flight on TAA, but actually took a tiny charter plane from Moorabbin airport. It might have been safer, but the unpressurised Piper Aztec took about three hours each way.

From Mascot airport, they took a convoy of cabs to the back entrance of 2GB. Sydney police didn't know that Dr Wainer had arrived until they heard him on air.

Then they rang and invited him to police HQ, but he made them come to 2GB. Mr Allan did not come himself, but sent Superintendent Donald Fergusson and Detective-Constable Roger Rogerson.

According to Dr Wainer's account, he went to hand Fergusson a sealed envelope with his information. The latter asked who his two friends were. When he heard they were journalists, Fergusson said it would be unethical to accept the information in their presence.

Dr Wainer replied: 'The only possible reason … is that you will be forced to act upon it. [If] I want to report a crime or a murder in Sydney, [do] I have to crawl into a wardrobe with a policeman and whisper it in his ear?'

The tension rose, Fergusson refused to budge, and the futile meeting ended.

Leaving 2GB, the visitors didn't risk ringing for cabs, but picked two at random. At the airport, Dr Wainer waited in the pilots' room. Then, steeling himself for the impact of a bullet, he forced himself to walk, not run, to the plane.

Despite the dangers, he did return to Sydney. In March 1970, Dr Wainer appeared on the current affairs television program *Four Corners*. In May, on another television program, prominent journalist Michael Willesee asked Chief Commissioner Allan if he believed there were abortionists operating in Sydney. When he said 'no' Willesee offered him Dr Wainer's list. When Mr Allan would not accept that, Willesee showed him films of an abortionist's surgery, reportedly within one block of police headquarters, then interviews with patients who had had abortions there.

Instead of receiving Dr Wainer's information in front of two journalists, Mr Allan had to do so in front of two million viewers.

New South Wales police then raided many abortionists, forcing Sydney women to turn to backyarders. As a result, more and more women came to public hospitals with severe infections from their abortions.

Police raided the Heatherbrae Clinic in the Sydney suburb of Bondi and charged the two owners and three doctors on ten counts of *unlawfully* using an instrument to procure a miscarriage. If found guilty, they could face 10 years in gaol. But the implication was that in some cases, procuring a miscarriage could be lawful.

In 1972, Mr Justice Aaron Levine in the Darlinghurst Court House, ruled that, for a guilty verdict, the Crown had to prove that a doctor did *not* reasonably believe the operation to be necessary for the woman's physical and mental health: 'The termination of pregnancy by competent use of instruments in the hands of medical practitioners is not an offence in this state.' This ruling reinforced the Menhennitt ruling of 1969 and drastically redefined key sections of the Crimes Act.

In 1986, in response to the liberalisation of abortion laws and their interpretation, Wainer said with surprise: 'Do you know what I am now? I'm almost respectable!'

He died of heart disease in January 1987. Friends organised what amounted to a state funeral; an opera singer sang

A Scottish Soldier. His close friend Evan Whitton called him 'the most extraordinary man I ever met'. In the eulogy, it was said:

> Dr Wainer's legacy to the people of Victoria from his great eight-year campaign was … a relatively uncorrupt [police] force, and the consequent failure of organised crime to get more than a toehold in this state. One's only regret must be that Dr Wainer did not happen to live in Sydney.

(GB)

3
Quacks, Pseudologists and Other Phonies

Quacks and charlatans

Generally speaking, the free interchange of ideas, the publication of new discoveries, the ready application of medical knowledge in sophisticated surroundings, and a commitment to aid the patient by sharing expertise, is the way in which modern medical practitioners go about their business.

Although you may occasionally feel that medical personnel are not always so virtuous, and can sometimes even be grasping, it is salutary to remember that in the past ethical standards have often been considerably lower. In fact, today's most rapacious practitioner has much to learn from some of his or her predecessors. So let us go back a couple of hundred years to look at some real phonies.

A charlatan is one who pretends to skills he or she does not possess, and the term is usually applied to the vendors of quack remedies who cover their ignorance in a spate of hifalutin and meaningless words. These people played on the gullibility and touching faith of the population, and for them 18th-century Europe was their high noon. Their advertising used jargon, classical or oriental names, intimation of royal patronage, claims of infallibility and 'secret formulations'. To compound the hard sell, there were usually unsubtle hints about the worthlessness of the opposition who, as one contemporary writer had it, commonly used his skill 'to influence the minds of the vulgar, or help especially those lately sporting in the garden of Venus and now tasting the bitter grapes'.

A good pictorial representation of such a person can be seen in William Hogarth's crowded drawing 'Southwark Fair'. He stands there, in laced hat and embroidered waistcoat, expanding on his cryptic skill. A written description comes from Samuel Curwen, who in 1781 travelled through London's Moorfields district (now the site of one of the most famous eye hospitals in the world) and came across such a character. He described the scene:

> A stage doctor on an elevated scaffold covered with a ragged blanket discoursing to the more dirty-faced ragged mob; demonstrating to their satisfaction no doubt, the superior excellence of his nostrums to those of the dispensary, and the more safe and secure state of patients under his management than hospitals and common receptacles of sick and wounded poor.

So the characteristics which seemed to set the quack apart from the journeyman apothecary of that era were secrecy, advertising, including dubious testimonials, the popular image of a care-lined pedagogue in declamatory pose gazing meaningfully at a retort of urine, and, above all, the skilful use of crowd psychology.

The purveyors of these impenetrable skills ranged from the simple market-day pedlar with his handbills and treatments for ruptures, VD and the like, to such as Dr Clark, 'sworn physician and oculist', as he wrote, 'to Charles II, James II and Queen Anne'. He advertised in top magazines offering his secret of 'the lamp of light', promising success where others had failed through the use of his infallible cure for the King's Evil (tuberculosis), cancers, and the stone (in the bladder) without recourse to cutting. No disease too trivial, no duke too poxy.

A less up-market practitioner was a Dr Cerf, 'lately arrived from France' who claimed to be:

> Well known for curing all kinds of disorders, both internal and external; likewise the SECRET DISEASE ... Trusses to be disposed of for all kinds of ruptures. Any person that cannot attend personally, by sending their morning urine, may be faithfully informed of their complaint, and receive such medicines as are proper for their disorder, on the most reasonable terms ... [There is] A back door with latch, by which persons may let themselves into the surgery. The doctor may be spoken with in all languages.

He sounds quite talented.

Dr Benjamin Thornbill of 'the orthodox city of Wells' (and few more orthodox than Wells, that's for sure) cured the lame, blind, deaf, and diseased, with dismissive ease. No possible pathological condition was regarded to be beyond his expertise.

Lengthy lists of treatable syndromes probably came about as a result of the welshing nature of the quacks' trade, in that they lacked those personal ties of reputation which the proper practitioner enjoyed within a neighbourhood. Mind you, proper practitioners were not above a bit of advertising to help retain an irresolute clientele. Besides stability, the local practitioners had two advantages over the itinerant quack: access to hospitals and the treatment of the poor and indigent for free.

The fly-by-night needed to concentrate on cures which were quick, could be confirmed at once by sight and background conversation, and conditions which did not recur before he or she had passed on to new pastures. The bizarre constituents of the nostrums added to their mystical quality, in itself part of the therapy. For instance, a concoction of snails mashed with bay leaves and mallows was advanced as a cure for the ague (malaria, then endemic in England) and a mixture of woodlice ground up with sugar and nutmeg was recommended for cancer. The juice of wild cucumber aided dropsy, and dung tea, stewed owls and crushed worms were given for a variety of complaints.

A Joanna Stevens was so jealous of her secret 'universal cure' it took an Act of Parliament and £5,000 from the Treasury to winkle it out of her. It turned out to be a mishmash of powdered snails, Alicante and other soap, calcined eggshells, wild-carrot seeds and honey.

Among other cures were Dr Belloste's pills for rheumatism advertised at a guinea a box and Parke's pills for the stone at 2s 6d a pill. Such a price would guarantee success: having been foolish enough to pay that, you would hardly admit to the cure's failure. Also sold, with equally spurious reputations, were Velno's vegetable syrup for venereal disease, Daffy's Elixir, Godfrey's Cordial, Scott's pills and Indian root.

Godfrey's Cordial was given to quieten fractious children, and very popular at London's Foundling Hospital. The snag was it contained laudanum (an opiate) and spirits, and its use resulted in numerous fatalities; a classic case of the treatment being infinitely worse than the complaint.

A favourite remedy of the time, and one which the writer Horace Walpole said would be the one thing he would rescue if his house was burning down, was Dr James's Antimonial Fever Powders. These were a combination of antimony oxide and phosphate of lead, a ferocious combination with a distinctly lethal potential. Nonetheless, the actor David Garrick gave a glowing testimonial recounting how the powders had cured his mother of severe hip pain.

This Dr Robert James was a qualified physician and had been at school with Samuel Johnson in Lichfield (Garrick's home town, too). He took to the bottle later in life, and it was said that he had been drunk every day for 20 years. He was damned by Johnson as a rascal after his improbable explanation for taking a whore about with him in his coach.

James's reason for such a coach companion was that 'he always took a swelling in his stones' if he abstained too long from sexual intercourse.

Despite his dubious lifestyle, he wrote a three-volume medical dictionary and was the inventor of perhaps the most popular patent medicine of his era. His pills were among many others which were used futilely to treat the mentally troubled George III.

Few were better at marketing themselves than another top-drawer charlatan, Chevalier Taylor. He claimed to be the 'sole master of nostrums and specifics in Nature, and the only oculist for the teeth in the universe'. You can bet he was. Doubtless he only dealt with the eyeteeth his clients would have given for a cure. As a result of his unabashed advertising, Taylor became one of the most widely known men in 18th-century England, even though Dr Samuel Johnson said of him, 'He is the most ignorant man I have ever met'—no doubt to be noticed at all by the old curmudgeon was a kind of reward in itself and grist to the publicity mill. Despite Johnson's riposte, or maybe because of it, he was appointed oculist to George II, George Frederic Handel and the eminent historian Edward Gibbon. Chevalier Taylor had his comeuppance in the end, for he himself became blind—but not before he had published a three-volume autobiography.

A contemporary of Chevalier was Joshua Ward, popularly known as Spot Ward on account of a birthmark on his face. He had started life as a footman, but obviously had his eye on higher things. Such was his influence in the court of George II that he was accorded official thanks by the House of Commons for his attention on the king, and granted the singular honour of being allowed to drive his carriage through St James's Park.

His famous Antimony Pill pepped up the likes of King George, Lord Chesterfield and Alexander Pope. Chesterfield was high on the social register, so that when he wrote Ward a fulsome testimonial, the quack was assured of a continuing and respected place in society. Mind you, the fact that Chesterfield was a vegetarian may have modified the action of the quite dangerous contents of the pill. Ward's Antimony Pills were in the same chancy category as Bateman's Pectoral Drops and Hill's Medicine for Mad-Dog's Bites—truly 'kill or cure' medicines.

One of the more interesting of these fashionable oddballs was Mrs Mapp, or Crazy Sal as she was known to her admiring and considerable clientele. She held court both at Epsom, outside the city of London, and in the Grecian Coffee House in Devereux Court, just off the Strand and a favourite resort of Oliver Goldsmith. She was a bonesetter, as had been her father before her, and enjoyed in her time such a towering reputation that the town of Epsom actually paid her a hundred guineas a year to live there in order to attract people of quality to the borough. She was there in the 1730s, before the advent of what was to become the town's even bigger attraction, the Derby. This was first run in 1780.

She ran foul of the medical establishment, especially Percival Pott, of Pott's fracture fame and eminent surgeon at St Bartholomew's Hospital, no less. He was stung to write of her:

> ... the lowest labourer and the most exalted not only did not hesitate to believe implicitly the most extravagant assertions of an ignorant, illiberal, female savage, but even solicited her company, or at least seemed to enjoy her society.

It sounds as though he was feeling the competition.

Sal, cross-eyed and waving what looks like a humerus bone, together with Taylor and Ward, birthmark and all, can be seen making up the ghoulish back row in Hogarth's cartoon 'The Honourable Company of Undertakers'. In fairness, it should be pointed out that the majority of figures portrayed in the drawing, though pillars of the contemporary medical establishment, are made to look no less loathsome by the artist.

Perhaps the most remarkable practitioner of this tumultuous era, certainly the most celebrated, was a man who ran a glittering establishment in London. He didn't have to trail round the royal court or country fairs soliciting custom—clients came to him, and gladly. His name was James Graham.

In 1780 Graham established the so-called Temple of Love in fashionable Pall Mall. He allowed his fertile imagination to run riot in decorating this up-market bordello, a place which was allegedly dedicated to breathing life into the flagging libidos of aristocrats and the well-heeled, so that, he claimed, 'sexual intercourse became an urgent need rather than a passing fancy'. Or, to quote his handbill, which he had distributed by servants in splendid livery and gold laced cocked hats, those visiting his establishment would 'find the whole art of enjoying health and vigour of body and mind'.

Inside the Temple of Love, the customer found a conceit of ceiling mirrors, glass dragons breathing bogus fire, and suggestive drawings depicting the sexual athleticism to which his clientele aspired. To heighten the drama, scattered in the foyer as practical proof of the place's therapeutic worth, were discarded crutches, ear trumpets, eye glasses and wheelchairs. A popular feature of the establishment was the obvious presence of gossamer-clad nymphettes among the potted palms. Included among these lovelies is said to have been Emma Lyon, the future Lady Hamilton, posing as a Goddess of Health.

But its main claim to fame was the huge 'Celestial Bed', where was guaranteed a rip-roaring night of lusty satisfaction to the impotent and certain pregnancy to the infertile. Indeed, 'perfect' children were promised 'as even the barren must conceive when so powerfully agitated in the delights of love'.

Inscribed on the carved headboard was the legend: 'It is a sad thing if a rich man has no heir to his property.' You might think Graham could have done better than that, but perhaps if you were paying a hundred 18th-century pounds for a night of bliss (which you were), mottos chiselled on the woodwork would be about the last thing on your mind. The bed itself is said to have cost £60,000 and had a mirror-lined dome above, coloured sheets and a mattress 'filled with the strongest, most springy hair, produced at vast expense from the tails of English stallions'.

Despite all the hype, it came to pass, as day follows night, that Graham died in poverty in a lunatic asylum.

Why did people visit such charlatans? Well, they were not all clearly defined as such. There was no doubt about the difference between the itinerant pedlar in the marketplace and the MD of Oxford. But until the Apothecaries Act of 1815 and the Medical Registration Act of 1858, the term 'qualified medical practitioner' had no precise meaning or limits, and differences between quack and doctor were fuzzy. So the reasons for their popularity are complex.

For the poor, the fairground quack was available and cheap. But the wealthy and educated also flocked in droves to their favourite pseudologist. Did they have a positive faith in the seemingly magical procedures? Possibly, but it is more likely that they attended after regular medical men had failed with their admittedly pretty thin therapeutic armoury. They marketed themselves well, and the medicines they dispensed—which often contained brandy and opium—were very patient-acceptable. If none of the proffered concoctions, unadulterated or sinister, is going to do any good, then you might as well take the one which makes you at peace with the world. On the other hand, quacks would have poisoned quite a few with the large doses of antinomy and heavy metals which were commonly used.

Down the years those who function outside the main stream of medicine have had a popular appeal when orthodoxy seems to have faltered. According to where you stand, they have been described as effective and efficient, or vulgar and dangerous, or natural and harmless. Doctors complain that the mistakes of quacks are not given the same full glare of publicity from which they themselves suffer in similar circumstances. True enough, many quacks have proved to be grasping opportunists, but many have not; the same can be said of 'regular' doctors, for the division between the two is not always easily defined.

(JL)

Those who know water

Throughout time, people have used urine in various ingenious ways. They have studied it to diagnose illness, applied it as a salve and drunk it as a tonic.

In ancient Babylon, India and Egypt, healers assessed their patients by looking at their urine. So did the Sumerians, who called their doctors 'those who know water'.

In 1090, the Jerusalem Code decreed that any physician who didn't examine a patient's urine should be publicly whipped.

At the medieval medical school of Salerno in Italy, uroscopy (inspecting and testing urine) went to astonishing lengths, including the degree of urine's concentration, its colour and smell, whether it was transparent or cloudy, and so on.

The urine flask or *matula* became the badge of physicians. In fact, paintings of Cosmas and Damian, the patron saints of physicians, often show them with a *matula*.

Some famous physicians depended on uroscopy so much that they treated patients without seeing them. Charlatans naturally followed suit. Calling themselves water-casters, water-diviners, urinarians or even doctors of urine, they flourished in most of Europe. Critics called them piss-prophets.

Many charlatans had an assistant chat up patients in the waiting-room. Behind a thin wall with a peep-hole the piss prophet himself would listen. Then he would leave the house quietly by the back and come bustling in the front door. Now he could simply glance at a specimen and tell patients that their husband had back pains, or that their mistress was pregnant.

Other assistants marked the flasks with codes for their master to read.

Some patients had tricks of their own. In the 10th century, Duke Henry of Bavaria sent urine from a pregnant woman to a Swiss uroscopist for testing, saying it was his own. But there were no flies on this piss-prophet (also monk and physician), for Notken tested it and declared: 'God is about to produce a miracle, for within 30 days, our Duke will be suckling a child born of his own belly.'

In London, the College of Physicians condemned those practising uroscopy without seeing the patient; a 16th-century statute also forbade the practice. But all to little effect.

One sceptic is on record as having sent a specimen of his gelding's urine which he purported was that of his wife. Unfortunately for the cynic, part of the quack's stock in trade was to keep himself informed on the ills of the district, and thus appear to have second sight at the psychological moment. So, having waxed eloquent about the lady's known gynaecological maladies, the quack concluded by saying: 'I grant that I may do your gelding good, if not your wife'.

A well-known uroscopist of the 18th century, at the high-water mark, so to speak, of such folderols, was Dr Theodor von Myersbach. He took up the art in the improbable circumstance of having been adjudged too short to be a rider in an equestrian circus. A doctorate of medicine was purchased at Erfurt in Germany and he was in business. Myersbach moved from place to place on the Continent, usually at night to be just one step ahead of the law, eventually to fetch up in London. There he rapidly acquired an up-market following, with such classy people as David Garrick and the Duke and Duchess of Richmond in his thrall.

His consulting rooms were in Berwick Street, Soho, and he charged half a guinea for a consultation. It must have been regarded as money well spent, for he is said to have seen up to 200 people a day. (They are the kind of numbers which can support a very large overdraft.) However, his carping detractors put this figure down to the fact that he had only charmed, rather than cured, hypochondriacal High Society ladies such as 'Lady Hysteric', 'Lady Credulous' and the 'Hon Miss Pregnant'. No doubt you can put up with a lot of hypochondria for 100 guineas a day.

He diagnosed by gazing at the subject's urine or allowing his hands to hover over the patient's body, crying: 'It's here, it's here,' when the vibes were right. Outstretched hands just about cover an average-sized abdomen, and if you move quickly enough you have a fair chance of being right, and in truth, 'it would be there'. Location of the trouble was followed by suitably vague diagnoses such as 'disorder of the womb' or 'slime in the blood'.

Suspicion was aroused concerning the effectiveness of his 'green drops', 'silver pills' and the like when a proper doctor, John Coakley Lettsom, detected poisoning in some of his own patients who had sneaked off to be treated by Myersbach. Analysis of the quack's prescriptions showed lead acetate in many, and in doses which would calm the colic all right, but only just before it killed the patient. Other medications were found to be water in which toast had been steeped—at least they would do no harm.

When Myersbach was presented with another sample of urine (actually port wine), he attributed the colour to a severely diseased uterus. The next specimen, cow's urine, showed 'too great a pleasure in women'.

Lettsom wrote pamphlets about what he described as 'this outbreak of urinomania', and sent letters to the Press to expose the charlatan. The public took sides, and a wearisome and vituperative slanging match unfolded. Myersbach upped sticks and returned to Germany, but he came back to London the following year and quickly regained his former popularity.

Indeed, it was because of such charlatans that uroscopy—which had been a respectable diagnostic procedure since ancient times—fell into disrepute, to be revived in the 20th century.

Over the centuries, many people have applied urine as a salve and even drunk it as a tonic.

Ancient Egyptian physicians treated sore eyes with the urine of a faithful wife. Chinese warriors would pause during battle to urinate on the wounds of their comrades to help them heal.

In ancient times, the fly agaric mushroom (*Amanita muscaria*) was a popular hallucinogen in Europe and Asia. Its active compound, muscarine, is passed unchanged in the urine. So poor people wanting to be 'as drunk and jovial as their betters' drank the urine of the rich.

The famous physician and anatomist Thomas Willis (1622-75) described the urine in diabetes as being 'wonderfully sweet as if it were imbued with Honey or Sugar.' Of course, he was tasting for the presence of diabetes, rather than advocating drinking it.

However, a standard 17th-century authority recommended several glasses of urine each morning for gout, bowel obstruction and hysterical vapours. People drank urine for 'Epilepsies, Vertigoes, Apoplexies, Convulsions, Lythargies, Migraine, Palsie, Lameness, and Numbness'.

Those with toothache rubbed it into their gums. It was also rubbed onto chilblains and chapped hands. Women drank it to restore their periods.

Russians used to sell urine to the French, who used it to make hormonal soaps and face-creams. A French dentist made a fortune selling urine as a mouthwash. Better still, he proclaimed, people rubbing it their body could lose lots of weight!

One Yorkshireman not only drank urine to cure his cancer, but also used it as an aftershave!

Early in the 20th century, a Mr J.W. Armstrong wrote a best seller, *The Water of Life*. He assured his readers that drinking urine could cure cancer, leukaemia, syphilis, nephritis, heart failure, malaria, swollen testicles, bedwetting, and even the common cold.

Clearly Mr Armstrong looked on the bright side of life. He found the taste of morning urine 'merely somewhat bitter and salty; not nearly as objectionable as, say, Epsom salts'.

(GB & JL)

Once despised and now revered

It would only be fair to mention a couple of practitioners who were regarded as quacks at the time, but who are now held in some esteem, if not reverence.

The Chamberlen family fell into this category. At the end of the 16th century Peter Chamberlen and his brother, also called Peter, invented the obstetrical forceps. The way in which the handles locked was kept a secret in the family for over 100 years. Because they would not share the mystery, and as one of the hallmarks of quackery is keeping knowledge to oneself, they were branded charlatans by their contempories. Eventually the secret was sold and the locking device was seen to be effective. Their invention came to be generally accepted by the medical profession and is used to this day.

The second family whose members were looked upon with some suspicion in their time was the Thomas family. In 1740 two small boys were washed ashore on the coast of Anglesey in North Wales. They were, it was said, the only survivors of a shipwreck. Both were adopted by a Mr Thomas. The elder boy, whom Mr Thomas named Evan, showed a singular aptitude for treating injured animals. That skill, plus the improbable story of his arrival, was enough to make the medical establishment purse their lips and wrinkle their noses in bristling disapproval.

However, it was this very same magical and mysterious aura which made the villagers take him to their collective bosom.

To cut a long story short, this healing gift, used in both animals and humans, was passed down through the generations. The grandson, also called Evan, spread his wings and settled in Liverpool to become the 'bonesetter of Crosshall Street' (later used as the name of a play about the family and presented in the 1950s).

Naturally he incurred the wrath of the local doctors, and three times in the 1840s Thomas was charged with neglecting a patient. On each occasion he was acquitted, the last time being carried from the court on the shoulders of a rapturous crowd, given a hero's dinner and presented with a testimonial. He was regarded as the saviour of the local dock workers, for they knew that if they landed in hospital with a broken limb they stood a good chance of it being amputated. If they went to Thomas, however, he would manipulate rather than amputate. His ability to set bones with consummate skill gained him considerable kudos among the less well-to-do.

Evan Thomas recognised, however, that the medical establishment was powerful, so he arranged that his three sons had a formal medical training. The eldest, Hugh Owen Thomas, was to emerge as the greatest of all the Thomases.

Hugh worked first with his father in the city of Liverpool and then as an osteopath in the dock area of the port. As time went on he became outspoken and a mite too forthright for the medical establishment. Although he obtained remarkable results in straightening and lengthening limbs, the medical establishment was very suspicious of the young upstart, for did he not fulfil one of the main criteria of a charlatan in that he was denigrating of others, especially doctors?

What the surgeons either did not realise, or, more likely, chose to ignore, was that he was one of their own, having qualified at University College Hospital, London, in 1857. He never had access to any hospital beds, yet managed to leave the profession two legacies, one of which is used to this day—the famous Thomas Splint for fractured legs. The other is the rather gruesome Thomas Wrench for straightening bones, and long since abandoned.

Hugh Owen Thomas died childless in 1891 aged 57, and although his funeral was attended by thousands, many in tears, it was not until years later that he was eventually recognised as the father of orthopaedic surgery, and one who had meta-morphosed the treatment of diseases of the joints.

Who can tell which of the eccentrics of today may not become pillars of the establishment tomorrow?

(JL)

4
Famous Patients

The mystery of Napoleon's Final Waterloo

The historian Hendrik van Loon described Napoleon Bonaparte as having an ego 'so great that he needed an entire planet … for his ambitions'. But when he died in 1821, he was in exile on the British colony of St Helena, a small island 200 kilometres west of Africa.

What killed him?

Napoleon's list of ailments reads like a hypochondriac's wish-list: epilepsy, migraine, relapsing fever (probably malaria), probable bladder stones, skin problems, stomach ulcer, under-active thyroid gland, pneumonia, insomnia, piles and attempted suicide! Some biographies also list chest and thigh wounds, though Dr Richard Gordon says Napoleon's only campaign wound was when his horse kicked him in the foot.

The French still argue that Napoleon's agonising piles were the sole reason for the delay that cost him victory at Waterloo in 1815. His opponent, the Duke of Wellington admitted: 'It was the most desperate business I ever was in … and never was so near being beat.'

Not only did the British win the battle, Napoleon threw himself at their mercy. But what to do with him?

Napoleon himself hoped to settle near London. Metternich suggested exile in the north of Scotland. The *Times* wanted to hang him.

Hanging might have been kinder than exile on the 'living tomb' of St Helena, where Napoleon lived out his remaining six years. Napoleon had 12 servants, 3 French officers and 3,000 British guards!

He kept up a flood of petty rows with Sir Hudson Lowe, who arrived as governor of the island in 1816. Napoleon was convinced that Lowe meant to kill him.

Napoleon became ill in 1817, with vomiting and diarrhoea. Dr Barry O'Meara, a naval surgeon, diagnosed tropical hepatitis (amoebic infection of the liver), which was common on the island. He wanted Napoleon moved, so in 1818 the authorities sacked him. The next doctor, John Stokoe, agreed with O'Meara, so they court-martialled him.

Then, by request of Napoleon's mother came a fellow Corsican, Dr Francesco Antommarchi. But the prisoner didn't do well. He still had vomiting and diarrhoea, and he was very ill for six weeks with a cough and with pain in his abdomen and shoulder. He was given calomel (chloride of mercury), but without benefit.

He was dizzy, so the doctor bled him.

By early 1821, he could no longer take solids. Still Dr Antommarchi called it hepatitis. While he was still alive, no one seemed to consider that Napoleon might have cancer, though his father had died of stomach cancer.

In March 1821, the vomiting was worse; by April it was black, suggesting internal bleeding. As he got worse they gave him more calomel.

Finally, on 5 May 1821, Napoleon died. He was 51 years old.

Six British doctors helped Dr Antommarchi with the autopsy. Since they could not agree, they wrote four separate reports. At first Dr Antommarchi reported cancer, but later he said hepatitis had killed Napoleon and blamed the British for exposing him to the dangerous climate of St Helena.

One of the British doctors also reported an enlarged liver consistent with hepatitis, but the governor pressured him into removing this from his report.

So did the former emperor die a natural death? He himself wrote in his will: 'I die before my time, murdered by the English …'

Over a century later, in the 1960s, there came to light several samples of hair said to belong to Napoleon. One sample reportedly showed that he had taken at least 40 doses of arsenic in his last few months of life.

In 1982, other researchers found that the emerald greens in 19th-century wallpaper contained a copper—arsenic pigment which a fungus could convert into arsenic vapour. They found a scrap of Napoleon's wallpaper which contained enough arsenic to make him ill, but not to kill him.

Some Frenchmen believe that he died of arsenic given over a long time, followed by cyanide. Others believe the confessions of Count de Montholon, aide-de-camp to Napoleon, who allegedly laced Napoleon's wine with daily doses of arsenic. Why? Because he believed that his wife was Napoleon's mistress.

So what or who killed Napoleon? Cancer? Hepatitis? The English? The wallpaper? Or the jealous husband?

(GB)

What killed Jane Austen?

Like its houses and its chairs and its coffee pots, social intercourse in 18th-century England has managed to convey to us a society which was at once both sensible and elegant. It seemed to manifest good manners, piety, and cultivated discernment—at least it did if you were of 'the gentry', which was the case with one of the greatest writers in the English language. Indeed, the lifestyle of the era provided the ideal ambience in which the genius of Jane Austen could flourish.

She was born in 1775, the daughter of a clergyman, and the seventh of eight children in a closely knit family. She lead a life of middle-class gentility and ease spent entirely in the quiet of rural southern England. Austen's characters and their backgrounds were drawn from her own circle, and they never strayed from the world in which she moved.

Furthermore, she was much too well-bred to let her own name grace the title page of her novels, and all her books were styled as being written 'By a Lady', as indeed they were. And yet her towering reputation is based on only six works of fiction published over a seven-year period. The first, *Sense and Sensibility*, appeared in 1811; the last, *Northanger Abbey* and *Persuasion*, were published posthumously in 1817 (dated 1818). They have never been out of print and have flourished even more since the mid-1980s.

Jane Austen was of a caring disposition and was the wit of the family. She never married, and it appears the creative impulse, then customarily fulfilled by the task of being wife and mother, was in her fulfilled through her art. She said her books were her children.

The author took considerable pains to conceal from friends and visitors the nature of her life's work and wrote on small pieces of paper, the more easily to slip under a blotter or into a drawer if chanced upon.

She led a sheltered life at home, interspersed with occasional visits to Bath to take the waters, or to London, or to the not too distant houses of her elder brothers.

It all sounds like a rural idyll, and so it was, until June 1816 when, at the age of 40, she had an attack of nausea and vomiting and low backache. It could have been something or nothing, but, in the light of subsequent events, was probably significant.

In July she was depressed and felt weak. This was put down to her dissatisfaction with the book *Persuasion*, which she had just completed. It may well have been, but two months later it was noted she tired more easily than had usually been the case, had uncharacteristic mood swings and further back pains. However, everything subsided and life progressed in its customary leisurely.

In December she declined an invitation to dinner using as an excuse that 'the walk is beyond my strength (though I am otherwise very well)'.

The following month she wrote to a friend that she was stronger but felt 'bile' was at the bottom of her general malaise. This may indicate a recurrence of her gastric upsets of nausea and vomiting.

All pretty vague so far, but then in March 1817 Jane wrote a letter to her favourite niece, Fanny, and in it gave the clue which could lead us to the likely diagnosis. She wrote: 'I certainly have not been well for many weeks ... I have a good deal of fever at times, but am considerably better now and recovering my looks a little, which have been ... black and white and every wrong colour ... Sickness is a dangerous indulgence at my time of life.'

Over the next two months she wrote to a friend recounting details of recurrent vomiting attacks, concluding: 'my chief sufferings were from feverish nights, weakness and languor'.

We know the slightly built Austen was bright-eyed and had an olive complexion, certainly not 'black and white and every wrong colour'. But a visitor in May later wrote that the author was looking very pale and spoke in a weak, low voice.

The family became concerned and moved her to Winchester to be nearer expert medical help. It was to be of no avail. Over a six-week period she became progressively weaker and had a number of fainting fits, until on 18 July 1817, after several hours of unconsciousness, Jane Austen died in the arms of her only sister, Cassandra.

So what did she have?

The story is one of unimpaired intellect but increasing languor, intermittent backache, fainting attacks, gastrointestinal disturbances, and fever, especially at night. Added to all that, and crucially, is a darkening of the face. The delicacy of the era regrettably precludes us from knowing about skin changes elsewhere, especially the vagina or in the mouth, or where pressure was applied to the skin (at the waist, for instance).

A number of conditions come to mind, but probably only one fits the whole scenario.

The lassitude could have been due to a rare neuromuscular condition, myasthenia gravis, but there seems to have been no speech or swallowing problems. Maybe the heart could be implicated in the form of bacterial endocarditis, an infection on the valves of the heart, but fainting crises are not known with this. Perhaps cancer of the stomach with resulting anaemia from the slight but persistent blood loss characteristic of the condition. Yet the digestive problems did not seem either very great or progressive.

Skin discolouration occurs in a number of general diseases: the rare so-called 'bronzed diabetes' or haemochromatosis, but the other symptoms do not fit; chronic inorganic arsenic poisoning with its raindrop pigmentation and abdominal symptoms, or indeed poisoning from any of the heavy metals, lead especially, and which could be ingested from medication or water pipes. But the other history is inappropriate, and no other family members were affected.

Pellagra, an ailment caused by a deficiency of the vitamin niacin, could be a long shot with its diarrhoea, dermatitis and dementia; but her diet was good and she was certainly not demented.

No! None of these seem right. From the records and the fact she was a country person with ready access to probably tubercular-contaminated milk, the most likely diagnosis is Addison's Disease due to tuberculosis of the hormone-producing adrenal gland.

Thomas Addison only graduated two years before the death of Miss Austen, and it was not until 1848 that he first described the disease which bears his name. Its best known feature is the skin discolouration, which Addison described as 'smoky or various tints of deep amber or chestnut brown'.

With the medical knowledge of his era, Addison was unaware that the blood pressure is lowered in this malady, for he had no means of measuring it.

Until the mid-20th century tuberculosis was the prime cause of Addison's Disease. Now it is likely to be due to an auto-immune reaction, as was the case in that other famous sufferer, John F. Kennedy.

Only one aspect does not completely fit. It is said that tubercular patients are commonly more sexually charged than the general run of the population, possibly due to the persistent low-grade fever. No hint of sexual impropriety in Miss Austen has come down to us.

Due to an overall lack of surviving correspondence, Jane Austen's biographers have an incomplete picture of what her day-to-day life was really like, either in sickness or in health. But we all know from her books that she was a consummate writer whose genius was tempered with gentle humour and a subtle insight into the moral nature of humankind.

It is better we remember her thus, rather than someone suffering from an uncommon and debilitating medical disorder.

(JL)

A medical history of Oscar Wilde

Oscar Wilde was born in 1854, the second of three children of Sir William and Lady Jane Wilde of Dublin. Sir William was an ophthalmic surgeon, editor of the *Dublin Journal of Medical Science*, a writer on Irish superstitions and defendant in an alleged rape-under-anaesthetic case. He lost, but only a farthing in damages was awarded against him.

Lady Wilde was a noted poet, and wrote a book on ancient cures and charms of Ireland. So Oscar was well-connected, medically.

The first serious illness of the author was in 1877 while he was at Oxford. He contracted what he called 'a positive sin', a Victorian euphemism for syphilis.

Due to the coy attitudes of the era, apart from that comment, diagnosis is based on circumstantial evidence only. For instance, we know he was given mercury, the contemporary treatment for luetic (syphilitic) disease, and statements by close friends at his death and a doctor's certificate at that time seem to indicate the pathology. Furthermore, he broke off a promising liaison with a young lady following advice that he should not marry until two years after the primary episode. There seems to have been no obvious signs of infection (such as skin lesions) during his life, and the diagnosis remains conjectural.

The only obvious effect of the mercury was that it turned his slightly protrusive teeth black, and thereafter he usually covered his mouth while talking.

If the diagnosis of syphilis was genuine, there was certainly no long-term effect on his mental capacity. He took the university by storm, turning Victorian Oxford into Periclean Athens with his repartee and well-honed English. He was awarded a rare double first in Greats (Roman and Greek history, literature and philosophy) at his graduation from Magdalen College, he won the prestigious Newdigate Prize for poetry, and all his life was renowned for the brilliance of his wit.

In the early 1880s Wilde easily established himself in the social and artistic circles of London by his flamboyant presence. The publication of his poems in 1881 was followed by a lecture tour of America. He hardly endeared himself when on arrival in New York he announced: 'I have nothing to declare but my genius.'

But America left one legacy: he contracted malaria, which he described as an 'aesthetic disease'. He must have had repeated bouts, as quinine was found in his effects when he was arrested 13 years later.

Wilde married Constance Lloyd in 1884, and by 1886 they had two children, Cyril and Vyvyan. That year he met Robert Ross, 'with the face of Puck', and they became lovers.

He had no intention of giving up his wife, but had to find an excuse to live apart sexually. It is conjectured by his well-regarded biographer, Richard Ellmann, that he told her about the syphilis and that celibacy was necessary. In any event, she suspected nothing, and sexual intercourse ceased.

In 1891 he formed an intimate friendship with Lord Alfred Douglas. This infuriated Douglas's father, the Marquess of Queensberry, who left an open card at the Albemarle Club, which said: 'To Oscar Wilde posing as a Somdomite'(sic).

In February 1895 Wilde sued the Marquess of Queensberry for libel, failed, and in April was arraigned for sodomy. He was tried twice, the first trial being aborted by a hung jury, despite the joyous evidence of blackmailing boys.

At the second trial in May he was found guilty and given two years' hard labour; a crushing blow for such a sensitive man.

At Pentonville Prison he was declared medically fit, so spent six hours a day on the demoralising treadmill, where he peddled mindlessly for 20 minutes then rested for five minutes, slept on bare boards and for the first three months had no communication with anyone on the outside.

The result was that he lost weight, became withdrawn and depressed, and suffered from insomnia. After some weeks, diarrhoea set in. As the prison lavatories could only be used during the hour of exercise, a tin bowl in his cell was his toilet. He was later to write that warders vomited at the indescribable sight that greeted them in the morning.

The prisoner fainted in chapel, and in the fall injured his ear so badly he spent two months in the infirmary. He was troubled by pain in the ear for the rest of his life.

Wilde was transferred to Reading Gaol. When discharged in May 1897 he was bankrupt, a social pariah and a broken man.

He went to live in France. There a persisted rash developed, possibly a vitamin deficiency—though he put it down to eating mussels—and he went to Rome to be blessed by the Pope. It did not help therapeutically, but of the event Wilde wrote mockingly to a friend: 'My walking stick shows signs of budding!'

Wilde deteriorated physically, and by September 1900 he had become bedridden. The skin rash was florid and his ear so painful that, according to a surviving bill, his doctor visited 68 times between September and December.

On 10 October, in his beggarly room, his ear was operated on, either to puncture the eardrum to let accumulated fluid escape or for removal of polyps. It was during one of the daily post-operative dressings he made his famous remark: 'I am dying beyond my means … My wallpaper and I are fighting a duel to the death. One or other of us has to go.'

On 29 October the ear developed an abscess. It was then his doctor lent credence to the syphilis story, by recording it as: 'a tertiary symptom of the infection he contracted when twenty'.

Morphine and chloral hydrate had no effect on the pain. On 27 November he became delirious and meningitis manifested itself. Neither ice packs to the head nor mustard plaster to the feet had any effect, and on 30 November 1900 Oscar Wilde died.

It is incredible to think it is only 100 years or so since a bunkered morality could cause such mental and physical suffering in trying to sanitise the actions and works of this towering genius.

(JL)

The death of V.I. Lenin

Among the side issues of the upheavals in Russia in the fairly recent past was the macabre rumour that the body of Vladimir Il'yich Ulyanov, better known as Lenin, was removed from its splendid glass-enclosed sarcophagus in the Kremlin wall and deposited elsewhere. Before he disappears completely from our consciousness, as well as our vision, let's just take a look at the drawn-out death and ghoulish preservation of the old revolutionary.

Ulyanov was born in 1870, the third of six children, one of whom, his eldest brother, was hanged for conspiracy in 1887. He adopted the pseudonym Lenin in 1901 during his clandestine party work after exile in Siberia. One grandfather was a physician and the other a serf, and he himself was regarded as a very bright student of Greek and Latin. But the fire he felt in his belly could not be fuelled by the classics, only by revolution, so he turned to politics.

His subsequent public life is well recorded; what we want to know are the medical aspects.

During the greater part of his life he was physically strong. This robust nature held him in good stead in August 1918 when, after an assassin fired two bullets into him, he made a speedy recovery, even though both missiles remained in the body. But early in 1922 at the young age of 52 Lenin became seriously ill with headaches, and in April his doctors thought it prudent to remove some of the ironmongery. He recovered, but in May had a stroke which left him partially paralysed and unable to speak. By dint of will power and a sterling constitution, the following month he recovered enough to throw himself into the formation of the nascent USSR.

In December he had another stoke with paralysis, and then on 10 March 1923 yet another cerebral haemorrhage which deprived him of his speech. It never returned, and he was in this hapless and, for him, surely most frustrating state until he died in the city of Gorki on 21 January 1924.

It was then there occurred an exacting post-mortem examination which in the end became a pathological *tour de force*, followed by preservation.

The autopsy was done by one man, Professor A.I. Abrikosov, but he had no less than eight top-flight pathologists and clinicians standing by, ready to purse their lips and suck their teeth at the slightest hint of hesitancy. Not only that, the Minister of Health himself was present, presumably to make sure the rites were enacted in an ideologically sound way. As reported in *Izvestiya* of 25 January 1924, it took three hours ten minutes to complete.

Externally, two old bullet scars were apparent, one in the left arm and the other over the right clavicle where the missile had been removed. The remaining bullet was found in the muscle covering the shoulder joint. The surface of the left hemisphere of the brain was depressed, and when cut open found to be extensively collapsed. Beneath the collapsed area were areas of yellow softening involving both white and grey matter, and cavities containing cloudy fluid. There were marked arteriosclerotic changes in the main arteries at the base of the brain. These arteries were considerably narrowed, as were their tributaries and the carotid arteries (the principal arteries on each side of the neck). In fact the left internal carotid was completely blocked. There was fresh blood in the mid-brain.

There were a few adhesions in the lungs and a healed scar in the left apex (the upper extremity of the lung, behind the first rib). The coronary arteries were narrowed, and fatty deposits were present in the aorta.

The cause of death was put as due to haemorrhage over the corpora quadrigemina area of the brain, and it was stressed that the post-mortem showed that most of the very severe brain damage must have been present for some time before death (a point perhaps lost on later generations).

It was decided to have the body lie in state. To this end it was soaked in the usual solution of formalin, glycerin, potassium iodide, alcohol and zinc chloride to preserve it for a matter of weeks only.

In six weeks some 100,000 people filed past, and there were many requests from outlying areas to hang on until they got there. Signs of deterioration with autolysis (cell and tissue degeneration) and skin desiccation began to set in, yet still the faithful filed reverentially past. It then dawned upon officials that the population of the USSR being what it was, this could go on until something pretty unpleasant was the only thing left. So they decided to embalm the body properly and display it in a specially built mausoleum in Red Square.

It was then that the embalmers received what they surely would consider *the* call of a lifetime, and the anatomy professor at Kharkov University was given the awesome task. Bit by bit every part of the body, including bones, was hydrated, depigmented with acids, peroxides and aldehydes, and then embalmed. Work proceeded day and night for four months, and the body was finally inspected by the appropriate committee on 26 July. It was declared to be sweet and, well, lifelike.

The Soviet Government wisely decided to publish the autopsy data at the time; political mileage might otherwise have been made out of it.

One bit was missing, however—the brain. It was hoped that its study by the renowned German neuropathologist Oskar Vogt would throw light on the alleged genius of its owner. In return for the honour, the Germans undertook to train Soviet scientists in their methods. A special institute was later built in Moscow, from which the Russians operated.

For three years the brain was scrutinised and picked over, until at last Vogt concluded that the pyramidal cells in Layer III of many cerebral areas were unduly numerous and large. At the time this was thought to have a mental association and was in tune with Lenin's intellect. More work was deemed necessary to compare the brain with those of other deceased intellectual giants, of which it seems they had 13 in stock. In addition, specimens from different ethnic groups were called for, as well as from some animals and children. A special questionnaire on Lenin's personality was devised, which was to be filled in by those who had known him.

And then, nothing; no articles, no huzzas, no Red Stars. The project was quietly, and probably mercifully, dropped. (After the Second World War the laboratory was found to be in ruins and containers with specimen brains and slides scattered over the floor. Nowhere was there any trace of Lenin's name.)

Vogt's study did not throw much more light on the alleged genius of the subject. There is no doubt about Vogt's diagnosis, but his ideas about the size of cells being of significance or that racial peculiarities affect intelligence were a bit outdated even then.

At least the team of embalmers did a good job. The old chief only needed to be dusted every now and again to maintain his pristine appearance which he held for over 67 years.

Where is Lenin's body now? Apparently it is still in the mausoleum in its original spot. The mausoleum was closed after the uprising of 1993 and the body disappeared from view for some time, but the building has been reopened on a very restricted timetable while the authorities ponder the sensitive issue of the final resting place of the old leader.

The Moscow Brain Institute, the child of the project, still stands as one of the leading neurological centres of the world. Perhaps they should bury Vladimir Il'yich Ulyanov there.

(JL)

Was Winston Churchill fit to rule?

It was [Churchill's] exhaustion of mind and body that accounts for much that is otherwise inexplicable in the last year of the war—for instance the deterioration in his relations with Roosevelt (Lord Moran)

Can we understand what drove a man as great as Winston Churchill (1874–1965)? Was it his parents' constant rejection of young Winston that made him strive so hard? At 18, he wrote to his mother: 'I can never do anything right. I suppose I shall go on being treated as "that boy" until I am 50 years old.' Or was it his belief that, like his father, he would die at the age of 46? What better goad to overachieve?

These were not his only burdens. Churchill was also unlucky in his choice of ancestors: five of the previous seven Dukes of Marlborough had had severe recurrent depression. Churchill himself called his recurrent moods of depression 'black dog'.

In 1915, at the time of Churchill's Dardanelles fiasco, his close friend, Lord Beaverbrook, wrote: 'What a creature of strange moods he is—always at the top of the wheel of confidence or at the bottom of an intense depression.' All this is very strong evidence that Churchill had what psychiatrists now call bipolar mood disorder (formerly known as manic-depressive disorder).

Even as a young man, Churchill was a health faddist, self medicator and lover of quack remedies. He used inhalations before speaking in public, and travelled with cylinders of oxygen.

When Britain declared war on Germany in September 1939, Churchill emerged from 10 years of political exile to become First Lord of the Admiralty.

In May 1940, after Germany invaded France, Belgium and Holland, Churchill succeeded Chamberlain as Prime Minister. He looked like Britain's only hope. Hitler had made (temporary) peace with Stalin and now controlled Europe; the United States still remained neutral.

But Churchill was now 65, and there were many concerns about his health. So in November 1940, Sir Charles Wilson (later Lord Moran) became Churchill's personal doctor.

This doctor-patient relationship continued, though not smoothly, until Churchill's death 25 years later.

In December 1941, at the White House, Churchill got chest pain. He said it was muscular but he was frightened; Moran thought it came from the heart. Luckily, it did not recur.

From early 1943, Churchill had several attacks of pneumonia. After meeting Roosevelt and Stalin at the Teheran Conference, he had pneumonia with heart problems.

Alanbrooke, Chief of the imperial General Staff, complained in March 1944: 'He seems quite incapable of concentrating for a few minutes on end, and keeps wandering continuously.'

At the Potsdam Conference, Churchill was too tired to read his briefing papers, and had to be carried in a chair.

The Labour landslide of July 1945 unexpectedly dumped the Conservatives. Churchill was depressed for months, but unfortunately stayed on as Leader of the Opposition.

A month later, after a long game of gin rummy, he had weakness of the right hand, but he recovered. Lord Beaverbrook made officials announce that it was 'a chill'. A Cabinet Office Under-Secretary, Sir George Mallaby, described Churchill at this time as rambling and lacking comprehension.

In October 1951 he narrowly won an election, and returned to Downing Street; he was now 76. Moran wrote: 'The old capacity for work had gone, and with it much of his self-confidence ... Everything had become an effort.'

For his fatigue, Churchill vainly consulted the osteopath Stephen Ward (who later led to the fall of a Conservative Government).

In early 1952, Churchill had a more serious stroke affecting his speech. By now, he insisted on even the most complex issues being condensed into one paragraph before he would consider them. Moreover, the Prime Minister often could not even follow a discussion.

Moran wrote: ' ... he was not doing his work. He did not want to be bothered by anything; he was living in the past ...'

But not once did Moran encourage Churchill to resign. Just the opposite:

> Winston ... once asked me whether he ought to have retired earlier ... I was, I think, alone in urging him to hang on, though I knew that he was hardly up to his job for at least a

year before he resigned office. His family and friends pressed him to retire; they feared that he might do something which would injure his reputation. I held that this was none of my business. I knew that he would feel that life was over when he resigned … It was my job as his doctor to postpone that day as long as I could.

In 1953, after an official dinner, Churchill had another stroke. This one affected his left side: he could neither speak nor leave the table. Again, officials hushed it up.

The neurologist Sir Russell Brain doubted whether Churchill would live another year, and agreed with Moran's view that immediate retirement might hasten death. A cardiologist was emphatic that Churchill could not act as Prime Minister.

But somehow, the wilful, wily old man defied such opinions, and carried on the pretence: instead of dealing with matters of state, Churchill read novels and played cards.

He himself once conceded that a prime minister could get to be past it, and should be removed, as Adam Sykes and Ian Sproat record in *The Wit of Sir Winston*: 'The office of Prime Minister is unique. If he trips he must be sustained; if he makes mistakes, they must be covered; if he sleeps he must not be wantonly disturbed; if he is no good he must be pole-axed.'

But there was no one strong enough to pole-axe Churchill.

In late 1954, he had to apologise after misleading the Commons (and jeopardising the government's foreign policy) about a telegram he claimed to have sent to Field-Marshal Montgomery during the war.

There was no such telegram; by now even the Conservatives had had enough. But it was April 1955 before the Prime Minister finally stepped down.

By then, he was spending most of his days in bed; his last years must have distressed those who had known him in better days. In January 1965, aged 90, Churchill died.

Details of Churchill's poor health did not reach the public until 1966, when Moran published his book *Winston Churchill: The Struggle For Survival*. Uproar! Churchill's family and many colleagues were indignant that Moran had revealed personal medical details.

But there is another issue, more important than that of confidentiality. Despite repeated evidence of Churchill's serious ill-health during the war, he did not resign as prime minister until 10 years after the war ended.

As Churchill's personal doctor, should not Moran have balanced his duty to his patient against the interests of his country? Could he have induced Churchill to step down earlier? Could anyone else have done so?

If we make pilots and bus drivers pass medical examinations, why don't we do the same for politicians?

(GB)

Josef Stalin and the doctors

Josef Vissarionovich Djugashvili was born in Georgia, Russia, in 1879. If he had retained that name he may well have lived and died a peasant. But he didn't, for in 1912, when he was invited by Lenin to join the Central Committee of the Bolshevik Party, he changed it to the Russian for 'man of steel'—Josef Stalin. It suited him well. Stalin was born into abject poverty, the son of a drunken, abusive father. As a child he endured a severe attack of smallpox which left his face permanently scarred. It was so disfigured that when he came to power, thousands of photographs had to be doctored to disguise the lesions.

At the age of 10 his left arm was injured, possibly as a result of being thrashed by his father. Osteomyelitis (inflammation of the bone) followed, and poor treatment led to a 'Volkmann's contracture' where the hand would not open fully and muscle control was lost. There also a permanent shortening of his left arm by about 7.5 centimetres. He often wore a glove, allegedly for rheumatism, but probably to conceal the defect in his hand. At times he also wore a brace on the arm, as can be seen in some unguarded photographed moments.

Despite these defects, Stalin was physically very strong as illustrated by the story that late in life he swung the beefy Marshall Tito off his feet in a bear hug.

But his violent upbringing had its effect, for as the years rolled by Stalin grew mentally unstable and more and more paranoid. He had thousands shot on the suspicion of plotting against him; his motorcade comprised five identical cars which changed position continually to confuse would-be assassins. In his apartment there were four rooms fitted out as bedrooms; not before retiring did he choose the one in which to sleep.

After the Second World War Stalin chose (or was forced) into partial retirement due to his high blood pressure, whereupon he became even more suspicious, calculating and irritable. Locks and bolts increased in number, and he had members of the Politburo eat with him every night so he knew where they were. All his food had to be tasted—and often had to be doubly tested—by his cronies.

By 1952 he was dosing himself with a variety of pills and iodine drops for unspecified symptoms. Though he had a physician, Stalin considered it far too dangerous to let him near.

And then out of the blue on 13 January 1953 the newspaper *Pravda* proclaimed that Stalin had uncovered a sinister medical conspiracy. It seems the dictator had received a letter from a Dr Lydia Timashuk in which she claimed Comrade Andrei Zhdanov and other Soviet luminaries had been poisoned by his (Stalin's) doctors. Zhdanov had been the party chief in Leningrad and freely canvassed as Stalin's successor.

But Georgy Malenkov, a prominent Communist Party official, also coveted the top post. In 1946 he had lost his job in the Party Secretariat following criticism by Zhdanov of his management of the dismantling of German industrial equipment and its transportation to the Soviet Union. So Zhdanov's death in 1948 was suspiciously providential as far as Malenkov was concerned. And indeed after Stalin's death he did become prime minister for a couple of years.

Following his old philosophy that 'if a report is 10 per cent true we should regard the entire report as fact', Stalin believed Timashuk's letter. Zhdanov had, of course, been treated by trusted Kremlin doctors who were well-known and respected in the medical as well as the political world.

The hint was enough. Nine were arrested and jailed for what came to be known as the 'Doctors' Plot'. Among those arrested was Stalin's personal physician of 20 years, Dr V.N. Vinogradov. He was arrested, beaten, manacled and committed to a dungeon on the suspicion of being a British spy.

Significantly, six of the nine arrested had Jewish surnames. It was said that five had worked for American intelligence through a Jewish organisation, and three were British agents. All were distinguished, but anti-Semitism was in the air.

More letters poured in purporting medical involvement in intrigue, and Stalin allowed the Press campaign to gain momentum. Members of the Presidium felt there was a lack of substance in the accusations, but never discussed it openly, because, as Khrushchev was to write later: 'once Stalin had made up his mind and started to deal with a problem, there wasn't anything to do'.

The interrogations began. Stalin was in a rage and, according to Khrushchev, berated the Minister of State Security to 'throw the doctors in chains, beat them to a pulp and grind them into powder'.

All the doctors confessed.

On 20 January 1953 Dr Timashuk was awarded the Order of Lenin.

On 1 March Stalin had a stroke. At first his fearful serv-ants were loath to disturb the apparently sleeping chief. When they realised what had happened, all hell broke loose and his room was packed with a host of doctors, politicians and security men.

However, there was no public announcement of any illness until three days later, on 4 March. Then Radio Moscow gave the news that Comrade Stalin had lost consciousness, was unable to speak and his right leg and arm were paralysed. Nine doctors were in attendance; a group of men who no doubt harboured very mixed feelings.

The communique added that the leader's treatment was under the constant surveillance of the Central Committee of the Communist Party and the Soviet Government. His chances of recovery were slim anyway, but such guidance would have snuffed out any hope.

Over the next few hours a wealth of medical detail was given to show that everything possible was being done: oxygen, camphor, caffeine, strophanthin and penicillin. Leeches were applied to his head. An artificial respirator was trundled in but, as nobody could work it, it lay idle as the patient slowly choked to death.

He died on 5 March 1953, aged 73.

A fully reported post-mortem absolved the attendant medical staff from blame. Nevertheless, of the nine doctors who signed the report, one died suddenly six weeks later and two others were removed from their posts and disappeared at about the same time.

The Doctors' Plot was Stalin's last purge. As no more doctors were arrested after 24 February, it has been postulated that from that date he himself was no longer directing affairs. It has been claimed the stroke was on that day and there was a power vacuum until 5 March.

It has been mooted that Stalin was murdered by poison and a battery of terrorised doctors went along with the lie. To support this it is pointed out that after the first bulletin the communiques became more woolly. For instance, it was said that the albumin and red blood-cell ratio in the urine was normal, but for either matter to be there at all is abnormal.

We shall never know if he was poisoned. We do know that Dr Timashuk's award was revoked on 4 April, a month after Stalin's death and the day the seven remaining doctors were ultimately released. Two had been tortured to death.

(JL)

Did a stand-in take the rap for Rudolf Hess?

... on May 10, 1941 ... the real Hess took off from Augsburg; a different man and a different plane reached Scotland. So much is certain. But the plot which achieved the substitution is still largely mysterious ... (Dr Hugh Thomas)

History tells us that Rudolf Hess became Hitler's deputy in Nazi Germany. On 10 May 1941, during the Second World War, Hess flew solo to Scotland—without Hitler's knowledge—apparently to offer Britain a peace proposal. While a prisoner of the British, he showed signs of mental instability. After the war, the international court at Nuremberg sentenced him to life imprisonment. In August 1987, at the age of 93, he hanged himself in Berlin's Spandau gaol.

But Welsh surgeon Dr Hugh Thomas agrees with Henry Ford who said 'history is bunk'. He argues that in 1941 it was 'an impostor who was thrust upon, or infiltrated by the British'. The real Rudolf Hess was shot down somewhere over the North Sea, perhaps on the orders of his rival, Heinrich Himmler. Moreover, the impostor did not hang himself in Spandau, but was murdered.

The following account is based on Dr Thomas's research.

A German pilot did land in Scotland on the night of 10 May 1941. He claimed to be Rudolf Hess, in search of peace. Though thinner than Hess, this man did resemble him. But it is hard to accept the 'confused and pathetic character' who landed in Scotland as Hitler's successor and designate, after Goëring. The pilot asked for talks with senior British officials, but knew little of international politics, or even of his own 'peace proposals'.

Prime Minister Winston Churchill did not announce the pilot's arrival, forbade any photos and kept him away from anyone who had known the real Hess.

Both Hitler and Goebbels announced that Hess was mentally unstable. Indeed, throughout his confinement over the remaining 46 years of his life, the prisoner's behaviour was puzzling and difficult. At times, he pleaded loss of memory; for the first 28 years, he refused visits from his wife or any other relative.

At the Nuremberg trials of 1945–46, the court sentenced twelve war criminals to death. Though the prisoner didn't seriously defend himself, he received only a life sentence.

By October 1972, when Dr Thomas joined the British Military Hospital in Berlin, the man known as 'Hess' was the only prisoner in Spandau.

Dr Thomas unearthed Rudolf Hess's old First World War records. In 1917, he had a gunshot wound which injured his lung, kept him in hospital for four months, made him breathless and ended his active service. But a medical report at Nuremberg in 1945 showed that the prisoner had no gunshot wounds.

During the time he had been a prisoner in Britain, Hess's British doctors had not believed his frequent complaints of stomach pains, but in Spandau, much later, he almost died of a perforated duodenal ulcer.

In 1973, the prisoner had stomach X-rays. When Hess was dressing again, Dr Thomas was close by, looking for a gunshot wound on his bare torso. But there was none. Nor did his chest X-rays show any lung damage.

One day in Spandau an officer called out for Hess. The prisoner answered: 'Sir, there is no such person as Hess here. But if you are looking for Convict Number 125, then I'm your man.'

In late July 1987, messages reached the Foreign Office in

London that a Soviet warder had reported the prisoner's 'loose talk'. Moreover, Soviet secretary Mikhail Gorbachev was pressing for his release, which the British privately opposed. The four powers controlling Spandau (USSR, Britain, France and USA) were to meet and decide this in late August 1987.

On 17 August the prisoner—by now very old and frail and in poor health—was resting in a garden shed after a walk. The American warder guarding him was called away to the phone in the main block.

The warder returned to find the prisoner's head propped against a folding chair. His face was purple, and round his neck was a length of flex. The warders could not revive him.

The British insisted that only their own military police should investigate the death and that only one of their own army pathologists (rather than an international panel) should do the autopsy. They also vetoed photos, fingerprinting and genetic testing of the body.

From this autopsy, Professor J.M. Cameron of the University of London concluded that death was not due to natural causes, but to asphyxia, compression of the neck and suspension. Moreover, contrary to Rudolf Hess's 1917 records, the prisoner had never been shot.

Though Cameron's report did not even suggest suicide, the British media release stated that Rudolf Hess had hung himself.

In outrage, the Hess family insisted on a second autopsy. Still no gunshot wound, but this second report stated that the prisoner had received a savage blow to the back of his head.

Finally, 26 German pathologists took nearly one year to compose a third autopsy report, which supported probable strangulation. Scotland Yard spent six months investigating the death, but British authorities suppressed its report.

Dr Thomas concludes that the prisoner was far too frail and stiff to have possibly hung himself. Instead he was struck on the head and then strangled. Furthermore, Thomas says, British authorities have continued this deception ('one of the most shameful crimes in history') ever since.

There is independent support for his views.

Seventy-six members of the Royal College of Surgeons of Edinburgh unanimously agreed that the prisoner who died in Spandau in 1987 could not have been the real Rudolf Hess.

(GB)

Kafka, Orwell, Camus and Auden

For many people 'the classics' are books they feel they ought to read, but somehow never do. This is especially true of the modern classics by, among others, Kafka, Orwell, Camus and Auden. Often these books are so tortuous that after the first few pages a reader feels he or she has the drift and puts them away for another occasion. For some, remembered books are the ones they have never read.

The authors are well-known enough, however, and a number of these moderns have had interesting medical histories.

Take Franz Kafka (1883–1924), for instance. Besides being the stimulus for a new word in the language—'kafkaesque', meaning 'man's bewilderment in a nightmarish world'— medically he had two claims to fame.

A thin, stooped, introspective man, at the age of 34 Kafka concluded that his then persistent cough was psychosomatic in origin, being initiated and stimulated, he felt, for the sole purpose of putting to an end his insoluble internal struggles. Being the reflective, introspective person he was, Kafka seems to have thought it necessary to have an explanation for every bodily function. In fact the cause was much more mundane—he had tuberculosis and was to spend half of his remaining six years in sanatoriums.

However, it was not so much the symptoms produced by the bacillus at its common location, the lung, which are of interest, but the symptoms produced from another, fairly uncommon, area for which he is best remembered medically. The germ affected the writer's larynx, and eventually left him speechless, parched and gaunt, a victim, he claimed, of a conspiracy of his own body.

Kafka's second connection with medicine was to do with his work. He lived in Prague and worked at his day job at the Worker's Accident Insurance Institute, where his task was to assess the degree of disability caused by workplace injuries.

He was there at a time when workers' compensation was an emerging feature of industrial life, and quickly recognised that it did not always pay to get well quickly; a clean bill of health often meant being sent away empty handed. Limbs became a commodity to be haggled over, and at night Kafka returned home to write about those more seedy aspects of human nature he had seen during the day.

Kafka always felt that he should have won the Nobel Prize for Literature. When it became obvious that was not going to happen, in a fit of gallows humour he exclaimed: 'At least I think I deserve the Nobel Prize for sputum.'

He was 40 when he died in 1924. Had he not succumbed then, a second fatal trap may have been sprung 20 years on, for his three sisters were gassed in a German concentration camp.

Another well-regarded modern writer was George Orwell (1903–50). He was born in Bengal, where his father was a minor civil-service official, and he grew up in an atmosphere of impoverished snobbery. Nonetheless, he was bright enough to win a scholarship to Eton.

Orwell was also to die of tuberculosis in a sanatorium. Furthermore, like Kafka, he had a laryngeal condition which affected his speech. It was not a chronic infection, however, but the result of a wound to the throat sustained during the Spanish Civil War. Thereafter he spoke in an odd, strained manner.

The Algerian writer Albert Camus (1913–60), who did manage to win the Nobel Prize for Literature, contracted tuberculosis at the age of 17. As a youth he rather fancied himself as a soccer player, but the disease cut short his promising sporting career. He had several flare-ups of the disease, but, as he lived on into the era of antibiotics, he survived with the aid of their use. In the end it did him little good for he died aged 46, not of a diseased chest, but of an automobile accident.

But of this small group of modern writers it is the poet, and one of the angry young men of literature of the 1930s, W.H. Auden (1907–73), who perhaps has the most interesting medical history.

He was born in York, where his father was a general practitioner (well-off enough to employ a coachman, two maids and a cook—those were the days). The year after Auden was born the family moved to Birmingham, where his father had been appointed to a post at the university's medical school.

Auden felt destined to be a poet from the age of 15, and his undergraduate days at Christ Church, Oxford, cemented his early aspirations.

Photographs taken in his youth show his rather florid face, thick lips and large hands and feet. Apparently he was clumsy in his movements, rather grubby in his personal habits and lived in an apartment which was to be avoided by the fastidious. He was described by Alan Bennett as: 'scattering his ash as liberally as he did his aperçus. If one wanted to entertain Auden, the first requirement was a good carpet sweeper'.

He was a professed homosexual and his long-time lover was Chester Kallman, an undistinguished young poet who apparently, as Bennett succinctly has it, 'went down on posterity but not to it'.

With Auden's heavy features and thick digits, at first glance he had the appearance of an acromegalic. Acromegaly is an uncommon malady caused by a pituitary disorder. Often the first signs of the disease are when the sufferer notices that his hats have become too small and dentures ill fitting.

In Auden's case, it was not until later in life, when he developed his famous creased, gouged and rumpled face, that the true diagnosis became apparent. He suffered not from acromegaly but from the rare Touraine-Solente-Golé syndrome, also known as pachydermoperiostosis. It is a very rare syndrome, but oddly enough it seems Racine, a towering French poet and dramatist of the 17th century, was similarly affected.

The condition apparently mainly attacks males and is an inherited developmental defect. It is characterised by clubbing of the fingers and toes, coarsening of the features, a rather lugubrious expression, oiliness of the skin and marked furrowing of the scalp. (The features can indeed be confused with acromegaly, however in that condition the facial skeleton, the jaw and skull as a whole are enlarged.)

There is no therapy. It is not fatal, and progresses for five to TEN years before becoming stable.

The ailment had no effect on Auden's capacity for work, and he lived to the age of 66, dying in Vienna in 1973.

His face, while not his fortune, was a constant source of wonderment to the public. After painting Auden's portrait, the renowned artist David Hockney surely had the final say when he remarked: 'I kept thinking, if his face looks like this, what must his balls look like?'

(JL)

5

Warfare and Medicine

Red jackets, tight trousers and cold steel: the medical aspects of the Battle of Waterloo

There was a sound of revelry by night.
And Belgium's capital had gather'd then
Her Beauty and her Chivalry, and bright
The lamps shone o'er fair women and brave men
(Lord Byron, Childe Harold's Pilgrimage)

Thus wrote Byron on the Duchess of Richmond's ball held on 15 June 1815, a function graced by the Duke of Wellington himself, no less, as well as 'a thousand hearts beating happily when Youth and Pleasure met to chase the glowing hours with flying-feet', to quote the poet. It was then, just when 'joy was unconfined' that 'was heard the cannon's opening roar' of the Battle of Waterloo.

It all happened a long time ago, when medical care of the casualties of war was quite different from that practised today. Sterility, antibiotics, anaesthetics and rapid evacuation are the norm for the 20th century. But what was it like then?

On 1 March 1815 Napoleon had landed near Antibes in the South of France, having escaped from Elba four days earlier.

Thus began the drama of the Hundred Days which reached its climax in Belgium, in the countryside just outside Brussels, near the hamlet of Waterloo.

During those three months the former Emperor had managed to gather around him 115,000 of France's finest troops, and on the very day of the Duchess's ball he quietly slipped over the river Sambre in the north east of that country, and, although he did not know it at the time, into military folklore. His plan was to drive a wedge between the 102,000 Anglo-Dutch-Belgium troops under Wellington and the 140,000 approaching Prussians under Marshal Blücher. Initially there was success and the Prussians were driven back to within 40 kilometres of Brussels.

Over the next three days several bloody battles were fought, culminating in the final showdown at Waterloo on 18 June. Many valorous stories are told of the brief campaign, but when the cannon fire had stopped and the smoke cleared, the chilling and sombre fact remained that all told there had been 102,000 fatal casualties including 47,000 at Waterloo itself. These latter were about equally divided between the two forces.

> And Ardennes waves above them her green leaves,
> Dewy with nature's tear-drops as they pass,
> Grieving, if aught inanimate e'er grieves,
> Over the unreturning brave—alas!

The question is: if Byron could thus verbalise the country's collective sorrow over the dead, how did the army deal with the daunting problem on the spot of those only marginally better off, the wounded? In a word: ingloriously. In deed and in fact, they had met their Waterloo.

The British Army medical department of the era fell into two categories, those who staffed hospitals, a phalanx of top medical brass led in this instance by Dr John Grant, who was headquartered in Brussels—and those attached to regiments, who were, indeed, at the cutting edge, in more ways than one.

For the Waterloo offensive there were 52 staff surgeons who were distributed among general hospitals at Ostend, Ghent and Bruges as well as Brussels.

In the field the theory was that each battalion of 600 men was allocated one regimental surgeon and two assistant surgeons. In fact, of the 40 battalions, only 22 had this complement. All told there were 36 regimental medical officers and 69 assistant surgeons in the action of June 1815. A veritable thin red line, with sleeves up and eyes down as the foot sloggers went pouring forth 'with impetuous speed, and swiftly forming in the ranks of war', to quote Byron again.

Assistant surgeons were unqualified apprentices and usually inexperienced in battle conditions The medical field station, such as it was, was often within cannon-shot range of the battle itself and established in a farmhouse or barn. It was expected to move with the action, leaving the more seriously wounded in the care of the local inhabitants. As the war had already ravished their land, a wounded pillager in their midst must have raised mixed feelings in the unwilling hosts. In the Waterloo campaign, however, most Belgians were generous, caring and unstinting in their efforts to aid the injured, after all they were actually on the side of the allies. Nonetheless, some went onto the field of battle when the combatants had departed and stripped the bodies of any marketable bric-a-brac. Moreover, to further that grisly end, they were not above dispatching a few of the badly wounded.

Between the front and the base hospital there were no intermediate units, but to overcome this deficiency, the authorities supplied each battalion of 600 with one sprung cart, some blankets and 12 stretchers. Brussels is about 19 kilometres from Waterloo, and in the end it proved to be a long and halting walk for many.

No operating instruments were provided, as each surgeon was required to bring along his own boxed set. These included items such as bullet forceps to grope for missiles, a punch to knock out teeth, a pair of strong flippers for trimming the ends of protruding bones and a probang. This later was a flexible strip of whalebone for rummaging about down the throat to clear the passages.

(Since this surgically gung-ho era, of course, such boxed sets of surgeons instruments have become collectors' items; so much so, in fact, that many extra assortments were manufactured to satisfy the ghoulish curiosity and morbid interest of the amateur collector. One seen now in mint condition probably never saw the inside of a field operating theatre or drew blood in the line of duty.)

The overwhelming size of their task at Waterloo concentrated the minds of the surgeons wonderfully, and the whiff of cordite and press of numbers rapidly overcame any hesitancy due to lack of formal qualifications or dexterity. For his pains, a Regimental Medical Officer was paid 10 shillings a day and in seniority ranked below the youngest ensign in the regiment.

Apart from three defended farms, the battle itself was fought over open country with little cover. This facilitated artillery fire and mass deployment of troops. As a consequence there were three modes of injury.

First, heavy macerating wounds from 6, 9 or 12 pound round shot. The allies had smaller cannon, but the French had the more deadly 12-pounder. The cannon fire was liable to produce violent effects up to about 1,000 metres, and a well-directed shot was capable of killing a dozen or more men in line. A ricochet could be just as lethal. Fortunately, the formalities that June day had been preceded by heavy rain, and the wet ground reduced the chance of ricochet.

Second, injuries from low-velocity lead musket fire. This was effective up to about 30 to 40 metres and the shot frequently fragmented on contact with bone. Over 250 metres it was little more than a nuisance, so muskets could only effectively be used at close quarters, which added a psychological dimension. Multiple shot exploding out of canisters was particularly effective against massed infantry.

And, if that was not enough, the third possible tribulation was of a cutting, chopping or piercing variety of injury from swords, lances or bayonets. This was very much the era of dash and elan, and the later recounting of tales of hand-to-hand fighting, especially if having taken place in scarlet jackets and tight trousers, was the stuff for romantic interludes in front parlours for years to come—if you lived, that is. You may recall Byron on 'Brunswick's fated chieftain' who:

> ... roused the vengeance blood alone could quell;
> He rush'd into the field, and, foremost fighting fell.

He was one of those felled on a tiny four-kilometre front. The Battle of Waterloo itself was the third and final encounter in the three days of the brief campaign, the exhausting culmination of a quite bloody frenzy.

It lasted just the one day, getting off to a late start at 11 a.m., when the muskets had dried out, and ending at sunset with the final defeat of the Old Imperial Guard. In that time the combatants managed to inflict 47,000 casualties on each other.

If wounded, but you survived, what would be your likely injury?

On the head and neck, chopping injuries were common, compound skull fractures frequent and death the rule. True, portions of the impacted bone were removed and skin flaps replaced, but the ensuing meningitis or cerebral abscesses with fits heralded the inevitable. There was the odd exception, of course, and he dined out on the story for years.

Penetration of the chest wall by ball or bayonet resulted in contaminated sucking wounds and drains had to be inserted. Your chances were pretty thin. It was thought at the time that if the man survived a glancing blow, any later onset of breathlessness was due to electricity from the passing ball. In fact, was almost certainly due to bleeding within the lung.

Abdominal wounds were also usually fatal. If the bowel was divided it was sutured to the abdominal wall in the vain hope of preventing contamination of the peritoneal cavity. A musket ball could lodge in the bowel and at least one soldier is recorded as having passed the shot by way of the rectum at a later date. It is to be hoped that the po-faced warrior kept it.

That leaves us with the limbs, and here, you will be glad to know, there was a glimmer of hope. Many tales are told of the survivors of chopping injuries and of those with limbs torn off. One sergeant rode upright the 19 kilometres to Brussels after his left arm had been torn off at the shoulder. He lived for another 43 years.

One famous limb injury occurred during the heat of battle. Cavalry leader Henry Paget (then Lord Uxbridge, and later to become the Marquess of Angelsey) was at the receiving end of a famous interchange while riding with the Duke of Wellington. It seems a cannon ball whistled just over the Iron Duke's horse and struck the knee of the disconcerted Paget riding by his side. Paget is reported to have suddenly looked down and said: 'I have lost my leg, by God.' To which Wellington replied: 'By God, have you?' He then turned and got on with running the battle.

The shattered leg was later removed under fire to complaints from Paget that the knife was blunt. But then he added that he had had a pretty good run and this would give the younger men a chance. (He was actually referring to the boudoir, not to the regiment.) Despite all his vicissitudes, Paget lived until the age of 86, and the wooden leg which saw him through all those years remains with the family to be still touched and marvelled over.

Surgical thinking at the time was that the surest way to save the life of a person with a compound fracture was to amputate, and the sooner the better. If left, sepsis, gangrene and tetanus could prove fatal. Incredibly, approximately 500 amputations were carried out during the period of the battle, and about

12 per cent of those a limb injury had the limb removed. No doubt many amputations were unnecessary, but hesitancy had no place with bullets flying about, so the motto was: 'when in doubt, amputate'. Mortality following immediate amputation was about 30 per cent, but if amputation was left until later at a base hospital, the deaths amounted to about 45 per cent due to fever and gangrene. So there was probably something in the clinical catch phrase, but either way you were pretty well on a hiding to nothing.

The actual operation was done by a kind of guillotine method and the skin edges brought together by sutures or tape. Speed of operation was the hallmark of the skilled practitioner and the drama took anything from a few minutes to quarter of an hour. As there were no anaesthetics available it must have been the longest few minutes in the man's life.

But in truth, it was not quite so bad as you would think, for the shattering nature of the injury had an important surgical consequence, which was not lost on the surgeons, even if the sufferer had his reservations. The blow numbed the limb and relaxed the muscles for a few centimetres above and below the injury, and as the blood pressure was low from shock, so bleeding was reduced. Another advantage of early operation, but not realised at the time, was that a dirty wound was converted into a relatively clean one which would travel and heal better. Further, it did not need dressing for several days and if the victim fell into the hands of itinerant sawbones keen to make a quick financial killing (if not one of any other sort), at least the operation had already been done by a skilled person. So carrying out surgery on the field of conflict could be defended.

Amputees were agreed that the most painful part was the skin incision and the clamping of the arteries together with their accompanying nerves. It was described as a powerful burning sensation. What they did not know was that it was better to be one of the early cases, while the knives were comparatively clean if not actually sterile.

Lord Fitzroy Somerset had the presence of mind to call for his arm to be brought back after amputation as he had forgotten to take off his signet ring. Another story for the boudoir. He later became Lord Raglan and lent his name to a type of sleeve which has no shoulder seams, the sleeve extending up to the neck, perhaps done to accommodate his injury. He lived for another 40 years.

Musket balls were probed for and removed and skin wounds brought together with either tape or sutures of waxed linen or twisted gut. The overall mortality of these procedures was about nine per cent.

Wounded men sometimes lay for days on the field of battle and occasionally for weeks in adjacent barns. For some survivors such a delay may have saved their limb, as there was some medical reticence about vigorously treating malodorous lesions.

For those who were picked up, the roads were choked with wounded making their way to Brussels, where six hospitals catered for about 2,500 wounded. The overflow of a similar number went on to Antwerp and beyond.

With the breaking of the news in England, many civilian surgeons journeyed to Belgium to help not only with the wounds but the gangrene, dysentery, and fulminating infections which were the inevitable consequence of most of the injuries.

However, not all things medical at Waterloo were of a traumatic nature. In his pursuit of Blücher, Napoleon uncharacteristically hesitated at what proved to be a crucial moment in the proceedings. He returned to his quarters and became preoccupied not with deep strategy, but with a pressing need to ease an acute attack of prolapsed piles. Having been in the saddle all day, doubtless he found this less than amusing. Indeed, the fact did not come to light until 50 or so years later when his servant, previously sworn to secrecy, told all. Ultimately, of course, his mundane lesion proved to have a more far-reaching importance than all the desperate surgical heroics being carried out at the same time all round Waterloo.

It is also said that the Little Corporal had a fit the night before the encounter, and his doctor left him to sleep in. He had had one previously, while locked in the arms of his mistress during a particularly strenuous sexual joust. On that occasion, the lady fled in hysterics when she feared her gyrations and excesses had killed the chief.

As it has been speculated that Napoleon died of cancer of the stomach six years later, his night before the battle may also have been disturbed by the odd twinge of indigestion too. It is not recorded.

The man who let Napoleon sleep in was his chief medical officer, Baron Dominique-Jean Larrey, and as he was the dominant medical figure in the otherwise oppressive military bravura of Waterloo. We ought to digress slightly and take a closer look at this remarkable man and his background.

Since the invention of the cannon and other gunpowder-propelled firearms in the 14th century, battles had become bigger and casualties numbered thousands rather than hundreds, or even tens.

With few exceptions, notably Ancient Rome, medical officers were not found in the army before the 18th century. Some went as servants to the nobility, but the rank and file looked after themselves, were tended by local inhabitants or treated by itinerant charlatans or camp followers. Logistically the wounded posed no real problem; they either tagged along with the baggage wagons as best they could, or were abandoned. Ambroise Pare in 1537 witnessed an old soldier calmly cut the throats of three men who were badly wounded; the old soldier then turned to Pare and said he hoped the same would happen to him if he were similarly wounded.

Queen Isabella of Spain (1451–1504) had provided bedded wagons to transport the wounded after the battle had passed.

The Duke of Wellington during the Peninsular War of 1804–14 thought bedded wagons a confounded nuisance and would allow nothing to interfere with the movements of his army. At that time French regulations stated that so-called ambulances should wait three miles to the rear. These were huge cumbersome vehicles known as *fourgons* and needing up to 40 horses to pull them. With the usual mud and road confusion, it could take 24 to 36 hours to reach the collection point to where the wounded had been manhandled, by which time those in need were either dead or in extremis. Many were left on the field to be swooped on by camp followers, stripped, robbed and mutilated; friend or foe it made no difference.

Someone was needed with medical skill and a will to stand up to military authority and get some order into caring for the wounded. Dominique-Jean Larrey was that man.

He was born in 1766 and joined the army as a medical officer in 1792. Besides his drive and enthusiasm, he had another crucial asset—he was a superb surgeon, a skill soon recognised by the highest authority. Larrey insisted on attending to the surgical needs of soldiers regardless of rank or nationality. For the era he displayed a quite unique humanity towards his fellow man.

At the beginning of his career he joined the army on the Rhine and chaffed at the rear. He thought he could get the wounded onto panniers slung on horses, but it proved to be impractical. The following year he sought out the commander, General Custine, and pointed out that while the infantry had the support of very mobile artillery, the same was not true for the wounded. He sought permission to construct a vehicle on similar lines to the gun carriages, and which he christened 'flying ambulances'.

Custine was a 50-year-old aristocrat; Larrey was a 26-year-old provincial doctor. Normally Larrey would have been sent packing with a flea in his ear for such a hare-brained scheme, but by significant chance the Terror was in full cry, and it struck the officer it would never do for the National Convention to learn that one of its generals had turned down a plan to help its citizens. So, amazingly, young Larrey got the nod.

The ambulance, Larrey insisted, had to be a carriage, well sprung and light. He got his wish, and each division was equipped with 12 carriages, eight with two wheels for use in flat country, the others with four wheels for mountainous terrain. The smaller carriage resembled an elongated cube with two small side windows and doors at each end. The floor was able to be slid out over four central rollers and was provided with a horsehair mattress and bolster. The side panels were padded for about 25 centimetres above the floor and four metal handles were set into the floor so they could be pulled out and used as stretchers. At 110 centimetres wide, it could take two patients at full length. It was drawn by two horses, one ridden.

The four-wheeled variety was longer and wider, though externally it looked similar. The floor was fixed, but the left side opened for almost its whole length by means of two sliding doors, so the wounded could be laid inside. It could accommodate four if they bent their legs slightly. A wheelbarrow was slung underneath to act as the forerunner of a trolley. The whole was drawn by four horses, two ridden.

Thus Larrey devised one of the greatest advances in emergency military medicine, initiating the principle of rapid evacuation of casualties which is still a cardinal rule today. It was a masterstroke.

Meanwhile, back at Waterloo, Larrey was actually in the French line during the final denouement and was observed at work by the commander of the enemy forces, the Duke of Wellington.

When told who it was, Wellington remarked: 'Tell them not to fire on him. Give the brave fellow time to pick up his wounded.' Then, wheeling his famous horse, Copenhagen, the commander-in-chief raised his hat in a distant greeting to the Frenchman, telling his aide: 'I salute this honour and loyalty you see yonder.' Then it was on with the slaughter.

The Waterloo campaign was a close-run military victory for the British and their allies, even the Iron Duke himself admitted as much. Drawn and haggard, Wellington rode through the field of battle the day after. It was littered with the dead, and he silently wept.

> The earth is cover'd thick with other clay,
> Which her own clay shall cover, heap'd and pent,
> Rider and horse,—friend, foe,—in one red burial blent!

It proved to be the bloodiest battle of Wellington's long career. During the action Wellington lost 29 per cent of his army, and out of his 63 commanders, 11 were killed and 24 wounded.

But, as Dr Haddy James, assistant surgeon to the Life Guards, had it:

> … was the real valour displayed more in the face of the enemy or by those who watched the long torture of bullet probing or saw the agony of an amputation, however swiftly performed, knowing that their turn was to come? Those who regained their native shores deserved the prayers and the ovation of the population.

As for Larrey, he became a confidant of Napoleon, was created a Baron and maintained a surgical dexterity until his old age. In his prime, his time for removing a leg—without anaesthetic, of course—was two minutes. At that speed, the fingers of any slow moving assistant would have been in danger, too. He died in 1842, aged 76.

(JL)

Florence Nightingale: nurses force their way into a man's world

My God! What is to become of me? I see nothing desirable but death (Florence Nightingale)

It was 1850 in Victorian England. The despairing young woman had money, position, beauty, brains and education, yet she wanted more. Florence Nightingale's mission was to serve God by serving others.

During her lifetime she was to fight and win a 'continual battle against officialdom, medical jealousy, incompetence and inertia', in the words of her biographer Elspeth Huxley. Before the nursing revolution that owed so much to her, nurses were drudges, famous for drinking and immorality. Doctors despised them, while some took advantage of them.

Overcoming family opposition, she prepared herself by visiting the best nursing schools and hospitals in Britain and Europe.

In 1854, when she was about to take charge of nursing at King's College Hospital in London, the Crimean War broke out. The British reached the Black Sea, but since there were too few transports to take them to the Crimean Peninsula, they had to leave their medical supplies behind. They could boost their spirits on the long crossing by looking out at the bloated bodies of their comrades—victims of cholera—bobbing in the water.

Many died before ever seeing battle; the victory at Alma brought more casualties. Care of the sick and wounded was hopeless. British war correspondent W.H. Russell's reports in *The Times* shocked Britain.

The ambulance men were retired veterans, themselves more likely to need nursing than to help others. Both medicine and warfare were still very much male domains. The military had quashed an earlier move to send female nurses, but by now Florence Nightingale's friends included the Secretary of State for War. At his invitation, she left England with 38 women 'ranging from Catholic nuns to drunken drabs'.

Both their welcome and their quarters were chilly. Before they could occupy their room, eight nurses had to remove the corpse of an enemy Russian general.

The water ration was just one pint per person per day. Food and medical supplies often didn't arrive; there were no cots, mattresses, bandages or tables, even for operations. Rats prowled everywhere, the hospital was filthy and the privies were blocked.

In charge of medical services was Dr John Hall, whom Nightingale called 'a fossil of pure Red Sandstone'. To his superiors he reported smugly: 'The whole hospital is on a very creditable footing and nothing is lacking.'

Hall's orders from Britain were to let the nurses enter the hospital, but the orders didn't state that the nurses should actually nurse! At first the doctors just boycotted the new arrivals. While they waited, Nightingale organised food, kitchens, bandages and linen.

In the first half-hour of the futile Charge of the Light Brigade at Balaclava, two-thirds of the British cavalry were killed or wounded. According to Huxley:

> [To reach hospital, the wounded had to survive] eight days' passage across the Black Sea ... in ill-equipped vessels, rolling about the open decks, often without drugs, dressings or even blankets. Then ... crossing the Bosporus in Turkish caiques ... to be dumped down in the stinking corridors of the two hospitals at Scutari.

To cope with the flood of wounded men, the doctors finally had to admit the nurses.

Operations took place in the wards. Dr Hall opposed the use of chloroform anaesthesia, but luckily his colleagues were more humane. Florence Nightingale wrote:

One poor fellow, exhausted with haemorrhage, has his leg amputated as a last hope, and dies ten minutes after ... The mortality of the operations is frightful. We have Erysipelas [infection and fever] We now have four miles of beds, and not eighteen inches apart.

By late 1855, nearly three-quarters of the British army were under medical treatment and unfit for duty. Most were not wounded but sick: malnutrition, scurvy, cholera and dysentery were rife. In winter, the cold steel of their weapons could bring on frostbite.

Within three weeks, four of the surgeons died. Despite a severe attack of 'Crimean fever', Nightingale herself visited the front three times.

Long before the discoveries of Koch, Pasteur and Lister, she fought infection with cleanliness and fresh air. Under the hospital lay a blocked sewer. Her pressure forced the authorities in London to send a Sanitary Commission led by Dr John Sutherland. They had the sewer cleared and flushed; they removed a horse's carcass contaminating the water; from the courtyard they cleared 26 other dead animals.

Dr Sutherland, a pioneer in public health, became her lifelong adviser, disciple and willing slave.

By the summer of 1855, the death rate had dropped from 42 per cent to 2 per cent!

Back in England, Florence never regained her health and could not travel again. Yet for her remaining 56 years, she wrote, published and lobbied people in power to help various underprivileged groups.

Despite medical opposition, she raised £50,000 to found the Nightingale Home for Training Nurses at St Thomas's Hospital. Within 25 years, the bad old days of nursing were past. Better nursing care supported better medical care.

She died in 1910, at the age of 90. On her death, Lord Stanley, the former chairman of the Sanitary Commission said:

> No person ... within the past hundred years has voluntarily encountered dangers so imminent and undertaken offices so repulsive ... in a pure spirit of duty towards God and compassion for man.

(GB)

6
Discoveries and Diseases

Early dentistry was a health hazard

Toothache is as old as history. Skulls as far back as the Bronze Age show dental decay, including cavities from root abscesses.

Most sufferers of toothache had Hobson's choice: suffer agonising toothache, or submit to painful extractions, usually leading to toothless misery and hunger. Only a few could afford artificial teeth.

Tombs of the nobility in Tuscany dating from 700 BC have contained partial dentures, some of which were removable. The Roman poet Martial, writing in the 1st century AD, refers to teeth made of bone, ivory and even wood. 'Maxima has three teeth, all...of boxwood and as black as pitch.'

The Persian physician Rhazes (AD 850–923) was one of the first to recommend fillings, though the alum and mastic he used must have been too soft to last. The Italian university professor Arculanus (1412–84) was the first to refer to gold fillings.

In 15th-century England, the drawers of teeth included barber-surgeons (who also cut hair and let blood), apothecaries, chemists, country doctors, shoemakers and blacksmiths.

They all competed with impostors wearing teeth as necklaces or sewn onto their belts. At fairs and markets these impostors played loud music to drown the cries of their 'painless' extractions. A popular saying was 'to lie like a tooth-drawer'.

Though she said she had faced the Spanish Armada with 'the heart and stomach of a king', Queen Elizabeth I dreaded the pain of extraction. In 1578, according to John Strype, Elizabeth passed 'whole Nights without taking any Rest ... her Physicians were consulted ... pulling it [the tooth] out was esteemed by all the safest way ... to which the Queen was very averse.'

Finally the Bishop of London had to set her a personal example, even though 'he were an old man, and had not many teeth to spare ... She was hereby encouraged to submit to the Operation herself.'

Later, Elizabeth used to pad out her unsupported lips with rolls of cloth.

Hogarth's paintings show even young adults with few teeth. Until the end of the 19th century, some people had to crush their food with masticators (like large nut-crackers).

Dentures made of ivory or bone soon blackened and decayed; halitosis made outcasts of their wearers.

In the 1790s, Nicholas Dubois de Chemant fitted false teeth made in one solid piece of shiny, decay-proof porcelain. Later, Chemant worked in England with Wedgwood porcelain paste, claiming among his many happy clients Dr Edward Jenner, whom we honour for introducing vaccination against smallpox.

In the late 18th century, tooth transplants became trendy; many poor people offering their teeth for sale. The heroine of *Les Miserables* had to sell first her hair, then her front teeth and finally her virtue.

Anatomist-surgeon John Hunter, whose 1770s treatise *The Natural History of Human Teeth* revolutionised dentistry, advised operators to line up several donors. If the first donor's tooth did not fit, try the next, and so on. After getting a reasonable fit, tie the transplanted tooth to the adjacent ones. If all went well, the teeth would settle down in a month or two and remain firm for three-to-five years.

But sceptics claimed that 'transplantings' were actually replantings; that the operator simply repaired the extracted bad tooth and put it back again!

Live donors offered single teeth for transplants, but for dentures, dead donors were just as good. Even a badly decomposed corpse had valuable front teeth; a single burial vault could yield teeth worth 20 to 30 pounds—a fortune in the 1700s.

A supplier told Hunter's pupil Sir Astley Cooper: 'Oh, Sir, only let there be a battle and there'll be no want of teeth. I'll draw them as fast as the men are knocked down.'

Many people wore dentures containing teeth taken from young men slain at Waterloo. This was before the days of disinfectants, but perhaps some people boiled the teeth before recycling them!

The first satisfactory dental cement (a zinc oxyphosphate) appeared in 1869. Soon after came the dentist's drill, and a wax for taking impressions.

Now permanent repairs became possible, but at first, filling of roots involved contamination with germs. As Dr Bremner says, in his *Story of Dentistry*: 'Frequently the teeth under the well-constructed bridges would abscess and develop pus-discharging fistulae, but few dentists were disturbed.' It was the patients who were disturbed.

In 1911, a London physician, Dr William Hunter, saw several patients with puzzling ailments. Some had had extensive restoration work (contemptuously called 'American dentistry') that was dirty and showed unhealthy roots. The media added fuel to the flames of dissent. Describing the bridges as 'mausoleums of gold over a mass of sepsis', Dr Hunter suggested removing the bridges and the roots holding them. Of the few patients who agreed to having their bridges and underlying roots removed, quite a number found their ailments improved.

Doctors started thinking about the links between teeth, gums and the bloodstream. They felt that a tooth abscess may spread infection to other parts of the body. That was well and good, but some doctors blamed teeth for any puzzling illness. Patients indiscriminately had their teeth pulled, their mouths wrecked and their faces disfigured, and often without improvement to their health.

Eventually, X-rays saved the day by showing which teeth did warrant removal.

Over the centuries, poorly fitting, insecure dentures have caused untold misery. Not only could they slip out in company, but they often hindered eating!

In Parliament Benjamin Disraeli tormented poor Lord Palmerston, saying: '[His dentures] would fall out of his mouth when speaking if he did not hesitate and halt so … '

Even in late Victorian England, refined women often ate alone in their bedrooms. Then they would replace their dentures to sit elegantly at dinner, seemingly living on thin air.

A dentist fitted a fashionable lady with a partial row of human teeth mounted on ivory. Four years later, she returned with a very sore mouth, and her new teeth solidly fixed with tartar to her own—she had never removed her false teeth, lest her family know her secret.

During a world cruise Ulysses Grant, president of the United States from 1869 to 1877, lost his teeth overboard; after which he gave up public speaking.

But a sailor visiting the Solomon Islands met a far worse fate. He avoided being eaten by cannibals, only to see his false teeth fall overboard; when he jumped in after them, the sharks ate him.

(GB)

The mystery of Mawson's Antarctic disease

A man from Australia, one from Switzerland, and one from England. Not an ethnic joke, but the Far-Eastern Sledge Team. It was part of the 1911–14 Australasian Antarctic Expedition, set up to explore that part of Antarctica closest to Australia.

Douglas Mawson, Australian explorer, geologist and physicist was leader of this sledge team and of the whole expedition. He was 30 years old, and had already spent two years with Ernest Shackleton's 'Farthest South' expedition in 1908–09.

Of the six sledge teams, Mawson's had the farthest to go. His companions were the 28-year-old ski champion—mountaineer Xavier Mertz and 22-year-old Lieutenant Ninnis of the Royal Inniskilling Fusiliers.

Mawson, Mertz and Ninnis left the Commonwealth Bay base camp on 10 November 1912. They had 17 husky dogs hauling three sledges, each about 3.5 metres long; their load was over 770 kilos. On days, they covered up to 30 kilometres. But often gales up to 120 kilometres per hour stopped them from marching at all.

Ninnis suffered a bout of snow-blindness, and then an agonising finger abscess, which Mawson lanced with a pocket knife.

By 14 December they had abandoned one sled after using its supplies. Mertz was singing cheerfully while leading on skis, with Mawson second, riding one sled. Suddenly Mertz stopped singing and held up one stock to signal a crevasse. Mawson called a warning to Ninnis in the rear and went on.

A little later, Mertz and Mawson looked back, but they could see no trace of Ninnis, his dogs or his sled! Where Mertz had signalled a crevasse, there was now a gaping hole, over three metres wide.

Secured by a rope, Mawson leaned out over the edge. Well out of reach, on a ledge 45 metres below, he could see only two dogs, the tent and food packs. Below the ledge, nothing but darkness. Could Ninnis somehow still be alive? They took turns to hang over the edge and call him. But after three hours, they could hope no longer.

Mawson and Mertz had lost not only their companion, but the main sled, most of their food, supplies and equipment, as well as the stronger dogs. They were 500 kilometres from base. The only hope was to supplement their food by eating the dogs. They killed and skinned the weakest dog, but the meat was stringy. Mawson wrote in his diary: 'It was a happy relief when the liver appeared ... ' Nothing went to waste. They made themselves soup from old food bags, and threw the dogs old rawhide straps and gloves to gnaw on.

Soon Mawson got snow-blindness and had to march with one eye bandaged.

On Christmas Day, still 250 kilometres from base camp, they were already down to their last live dog.

On New Year's Eve the usually cheerful Mertz was silent. He thought the dog meat was upsetting him, so they agreed not to eat it for a few days. The next day, both had stomach pains and peeling skin.

On 3 January Mertz got frostbite of the fingers, followed by diarrhoea; they covered only seven kilometres. The weather the next day was fine, but Mertz could not march at all; nor the day after.

On 6 January Mawson, though he himself felt weak and dizzy, rigged up a sail on the sled and dragged Mertz along.

When they camped, Mertz had vomiting and diarrhoea; that night, he was incontinent. In the morning, he had some kind of fit. Then delirium, more incontinence and more fits; his violent movements broke a tent-pole.

Mawson wrote: 'I cannot leave him ... It is very hard for me—to be within 160 kilometres of the hut [base camp] ... both our chances are going now.'

During the night of 7 January, Mertz died quietly in his sleep. Two old sledge-runners became his cross.

Mawson himself had still had severe stomach pains and persistent sores on his fingers. Several toes were blackening and festering. When the skin peeled off his feet, he bandaged it back on as protection. He wrote: 'My whole body is ... rotting ... frostbitten fingertips, festerings ... skin coming off whole body.'

On 14 January, while he was pulling the sledge with a rope, a bridge of snow collapsed under him. Mawson found himself dangling four metres down another crevasse. As the sled kept sliding towards the edge, the rope supporting him was slipping. At last, it caught hold in the snow. Reprieved for the moment, Mawson worked his way up the knotted rope. He had forced his head and shoulders up over the edge, when the snow gave way, but then caught hold again. He fell a second time, coming to rest even further down; one finger was now injured. Somehow Mawson forced himself up once more.

Before setting out again, he made a rope ladder, attaching one end to his harness and the other to the sled. The next time he plunged into a crevasse, Mawson was able to climb out.

Blizzards pinned him down for days on end. Mawson had to open a boil on his leg; his feet were getting worse.

On 24 January he wrote: 'Both my hands have shed the skin in large sheets ... ' Next day, deep snowfalls squashed the tent until it was no bigger than a coffin; a gloomy thought. By now he was overdue at base camp. On 26 January he pushed himself in high winds for 13 kilometres, and then battled for two hours to get the tent up.

On 30 January he saw something black 300 metres north of his path; a cloth on snow-blocks. The relief party had left food and a note; he had missed them by just six hours!

For 46 days, Mawson had navigated with a damaged theodolite, a compass affected by the proximity of the South Magnetic Pole, and a watch that kept stopping. He had had to measure distances with a damaged sledge cyclometer. Yet here he was returning to base within 300 metres of his expected route!

Mawson reached base camp on 8 February 1913. He weighed only 48 kilograms; just over half his usual weight. His legs were swollen, he slept badly and had diarrhoea.

Even seven weeks later, Mawson's nerves were still bad, and he feared for his sanity. Luckily, his fears were groundless and he recovered.

Mawson received a knighthood and returned to lead the two voyages of the British, Australian and New Zealand Antarctic Research Expedition (BANZARE) of 1929–31.

His diary of 1913 described a condition that baffled scientists and doctors for the next 50 years. What strange disorder had killed Xavier Mertz and almost claimed Douglas Mawson as well?

They had suffered weakness and depression, loss of skin and hair, abdominal pain, diarrhoea, muscle and joint pain, nose-bleeds and swollen legs. Mertz had suffered delirium and fits.

There were clues to the diagnosis, not in medical journals, but from ancient tales of travellers and Eskimos.

Way back in 1609, Gerrit de Veer had written *The True and Perfect Description of Three Voyages so Strange and Wonderful the Like Hath Never Been Heard Before: The Navigation into the North Seas, etc.* This described Willem Barents's expedition of 1596, to find a northeast passage to Asia. When their ship became icebound, the party had to winter on the Arctic island of Novaya Zemlya. Hunger forced some of them to eat the liver of a polar bear:

> … the taste liked us well, but it made us all sicke … we verily thought that we should have lost them for all, their skins came off from foote to heade; but yet they recovered again …

In the 19th century, Arctic explorers who had eaten polar-bear liver described a similar disorder. Moreover, Eskimos did not eat polar-bear liver.

During the Second World War, studies of two polar-bear livers showed no poisons. But the concentration of Vitamin A was about 100 times that of ox or lamb liver.

Could polar-bear liver poisoning actually be Vitamin A toxicity?

The Norwegian scientist Dr Kaara Rodahl tried feeding the liver to rats, but most would not touch it. Only five ate any; three of these stayed well, one became ill, and one died. Experiments with extract of liver were inconclusive.

In 1947 Rodahl joined a Danish expedition to Greenland, where he collected livers of many Arctic animals. He found high concentrations of Vitamin A, not only in the liver of polar bears, but also in every Arctic animal whose liver was said to be poisonous. Conversely, animals like the walrus and Arctic hare, which the Eskimos said were safe, had low concentrations.

By the time Rodahl published his findings, preparations of Vitamin A were available. Some enthusiasts were overdosing themselves, and some doctors were also prescribing it.

The first cases of hypervitaminosis A in children were recognised in 1944; the first adult cases in 1951.

In 1969 Professor Sir John Cleland and Dr R.V. Southcott suggested that Mawson and Mertz had contracted hyper-vitaminosis A by eating the livers of husky dogs. Mertz's symptoms seemed to match the acute form, Mawson's the more chronic form.

In 1971 staff of the Australia National Antarctic Research Expedition (ANARE) collected the livers of husky dogs and found very high concentrations of Vitamin A: about 100 grams of husky liver contained a toxic dose.

But Sir Douglas Mawson could not share these findings. He had died in 1958.

Since 1959, the Mawson Institute of Antarctic Research in Adelaide has been carrying on his work.

Australia is also preserving physical reminders of the trials and successes of Mawson and his team. In the summer of 1997–98, a team of ten specialists repaired and conserved the huts that supported the 1911–14 Antarctic expeditions.

(GB)

Kuru and the cannibals

New Guinea, after Greenland the second largest island in the world, is Australia's nearest neighbour. The island is divided politically into two: the Indonesian province of Irian Jaya to the west, and Papua New Guinea to the east (which achieved its independence from Australia in 1975).

It was as recently as 1936 that the eastern highlands of New Guinea were first officially explored and gold prospector Ted Eubanks first came across the Fore people. The Fore were of short stature and lived in mainly an agricultural community where the men slept in a central lodge and the women and children in smaller peripheral huts. Strangers were treated with suspicion, and the Fore were not above a bit of cannibalism after a skirmish, to placate their fears of lurking sorcery and ghosts.

In December 1953, Mr J.R. MacArthur, a patrol officer in the Fore's region south of Kainantu, observed 'an unusual occurrence', as the jargon has it. He saw a small girl sitting by the fire shaking violently and jerking her head from side to side. He was told that she was a victim of sorcery and would die. The syndrome was called locally 'Kuru', which meant shaking, and was also the name given to a curse which condemned its victims to a sure death.

To inflict the curse, it was said, a journeyman sorcerer bound some of the victim's hair or clothing with a bundle of twigs and leaves, beat this with a stick while murmuring an incantation and then buried the whole. As it rotted, so the victim's health languished. A bemused MacArthur thought the effect psychological, even though it had come close to wiping out some villages.

The victim was usually a woman and the onset of the condition insidious. The gait was the first thing to be disturbed, to be followed by tremor and purposeless movements. Realisation that she had been struck down naturally made the sufferer nervous, almost paranoid, and she usually withdrew into the bush. Kinsfolk tried to identify the magician by a variety of well-tried methods; if someone was suspected strongly enough, he was waylaid and killed in a suitably grotesque manner.

The victim usually moved back to her hut, but eventually walking and even sitting upright became impossible. Weakness became profound and eventually the voice gave out. It took about two years to die a miserable death.

In 1955 a Government medical officer, Dr Vincent Zigas, discounted the sorcery mumbo jumbo and concluded that here was a hitherto undescribed organic lesion occurring in epidemic proportions. Specimens sent to the Walter and Eliza Hall Institute in Melbourne rendered up no clue as to the diagnosis.

An impasse had been reached, when out of the West came a knight in shining armour in the form of an American, Dr Carleton Gajdusek. He had been working under Sir Macfarlane Burnet in Melbourne but had never seen anything like this, even in Victoria. So with no official backing or resources he attempted to unravel the mystery. To not put too fine a point on it, there was some establishment resistance, including at first from Macfarlane Burnet himself. But in the end Macfarlane Burnet graciously deferred by saying he had an exasperated affection for Gajdusek, so gave him his full support.

The first thoughts were that the malady was a meningo encephalitis, an inflammation of the brain and its lining, but tests were negative. Anyway it did not seem to be infectious. No unrecognised toxic substance in common use could be implicated, nor could a dietary deficiency. The locals became dubious of the Western hype and not unreasonably suggested that examining the eyes with an ophthalmoscope may allow the viewer to catch sight of the sorcerer.

Gajdusek tracked down cases throughout the region and established that the current epidemic was fairly recent, and occurred in a circumscribed area being prevalent where the Fore people had made contact with their neighbours. As no white person had ever contracted Kuru, Gajdusek postulated that it was genetic in origin.

By now Kuru had made such inroads into the female population that the men began to move out. The Australian administration reasoned that if it was genetically spread, as was supposed, it could burgeon forth, so they placed the Fore people in quarantine.

There the situation bogged down in uneasy stalemate until in 1959 a veterinary scientist in a letter to the *Lancet* wondered aloud about the similarity between Kuru and scrapie, a disease of sheep. Symptoms were similar, but, as was pointed out, lab tests had already been carried out on animals and found to be negative. But they had only been sustained for a few weeks, even though it was known that if the brain cells of an infected sheep are injected into a healthy animal it will take two to three years to develop the condition.

With some reluctance at having to go over old ground, Gajdusek had specimens flown to America where they were injected into chimpanzees. That was in the summer of 1962. By late 1965 the first chimpanzees began to fall ill displaying all the signs of Kuru.

It was now obvious that the malady could not be genetic, and to cut a long story short, further examination located a virus with an incredibly long incubation period; in fact, a so-called 'slow virus'. Marvellous!

But why only in the Fore, and why mainly women?

Two anthropologists, Robert and Shirley Glasse, provided the last pieces in the jigsaw almost at once. They found that the first case had occurred in the early 20th century, and the spread, incredibly, was inexorably linked to cannibalism.

While cannibalism had been usual among other tribes in Papua New Guinea, it was relatively new to the Fore. Visiting the Kamano peoples in 1915 the Fore had seen it for the first time, thought how splendid the idea was, and took it to their bosom. So enthusiastic did the Fore feel about the habit that it became an important part of their funeral ritual. The whole of the dead relative's body was consumed and a pecking order developed, so to speak, clearly setting out who got which bit. For instance, the mother's brother's wife had first claim to the brain.

Two features emerged. First, as the men thought such activity would impair their fighting ability and so was to be regarded with circumspection, it was the women and children who had the lion's share. And second, insufficient cooking meant that germs were rarely destroyed.

As the incubation period for the slow virus is between two and twenty years, the victims had contracted the disease before the appearance of white people. With the stopping of cannibalism, Kuru should die out, which is proving to be the case.

So by the efforts of Carleton Gajdusek, the Fore people regained the harmony of their former lifestyle, and in 1976 Gajdusek gained the Nobel Prize for Medicine (with Baruch Blumberg).

Thomas Gray, if he had been alive, may have come from contemplating Eton College, looked at the Fore people instead, and then have written:

> Alas, regardless of their doom,
> The little victims play!
> No sense of ills to come,
> Nor care beyond today.
> Those in the deeper vitals rage:
> Poverty filled and tireless
> That numbs the soul with icy hand
> And slow consuming virus.

Swine Fever: the non-epidemic of 1976

Many of us have heard tell of the so-called 'Spanish flu' epidemic of 1918, and some will remember the 'Asian flu' pandemic of 1957 and the 'Hong Kong flu' of 1968. But not many will recall the 'swine flu' epidemic of 1976—this is perhaps hardly surprising, because it never happened.

In January 1976 at the American Army depot in Fort Dix, New Jersey, several soldiers became ill with a respiratory infection. Despite his fever, one foolhardy 19-year-old recruit went on an eight-kilometre march in the snow, then collapsed and died. Throat washings from him and four others identified two strains of influenza virus: A Victoria and another which the lab could not classify. If this proved to be a new breed of virus there could be no community immunity—the setting for an epidemic.

On 12 February the elusive culprit was identified as swine flu, so named because it was passed around pigs, but never before, it seemed, passed from human to human. However, it was for another reason that a few eyebrows were raised in the Centre for Disease Control (CDC) in Atlanta: the germ genetically resembled the virus which had caused the infamous 1918 Spanish flu epidemic during which 20 million people worldwide had died. It had never recurred, hence by 1976 nobody under the age of about 55 had any circulating antibodies. There was some high-level anxiety.

Two days later a medical conference of top brass was held where it was resolved to establish whether the infected four had had contact with pigs and if others were coming down with the fever. Was it the first rumblings of a pandemic?

Such imponderables are, of course, the breath of life to laboratory people, and they were exhilarated by the prospect of the heroic decisions that were to come. They were not to be disappointed.

At Fort Dix 77 soldiers were found to have swine flu antibodies, but were symptomless; 11 more were ill and positive. However, hundreds of others were in hospital with A Victoria flu alone. On the strength of these 11 it was concluded on 10 March that there was a '2 to 20 per cent' chance of a swine fever epidemic. There was division on the seriousness of the scenario, but the fact that there had been one death, plus the spectre of 1918 and the low immunity within the population helped shape conclusions. Less troubled pathologists felt the 1918 deaths were largely due to a now-treatable bacterial infection occurring on top of the virus. But either way, the epidemiologists sensed their day was at hand and a vaccine should be prepared.

That being agreed, the next question was, should there be a prompt inoculation of everybody, or should it be stockpiled to await developments? More acrimony. It was pointed out that with 200 million plus doses, even a small percentage reacting unfavourably amounted to a sizeable number of people. But Dr David Sencer, the CDC's director and a persuasive and respected scientist cum bureaucrat, was eager to proceed. He felt the vaccine was as 'safe as water' and the issue was one of 'lives versus dollars'. The price of the 213 million doses was put at $135 million.

Vigorous prodding by Sencer forced a dithering David Mathews, Secretary of State for Health, not only to grow in enthusiasm but also to find it politically attractive to say 'yes'. The watchdog of the country's fiscal arrangements was more stubborn, until it was pointed out that he was dealing with death and, above all, it was a presidential election year, with all that that implied. If a clincher was needed, that was it.

Gerald Ford was the incumbent in the White House, and was already seen as indecisive and bumbling: 'He couldn't walk and chew gum at the same time.' He tripped up aircraft steps and bounced golf balls off spectators' heads, but the swine fever program offered him a heaven-sent opportunity to transform his image. If a pandemic did come it would not only have been morally delinquent but politically suicidal not to have offered protection.

So, on 24 March 1976, flanked by Jonas Salk and Albert Sabin, of polio vaccine fame, President Ford launched the program to inoculate 'every one of my fellow Americans' against Swine fever. It was an unprecedented decision by an American president and at the time seemed a major triumph for preventative medicine. In the end it became a victim of Murphy's Law 'whatever can go wrong, will'.

Many public health workers thought the plan premature; no other country had such a scheme. Some said that 15 per cent would get side effects—about 30 million people. Money for other pressing health measures had to be diverted. Eggs for the culture became scarce. Swine fever was mild and not very contagious—none of the soldiers relatives seemed to have caught it. The dose for children was uncertain. And so on.

By June there had been no new cases and the Press was asking questions. As early as April the manufacturers had said they could not produce 200 million doses by the autumn, the ideal time for inoculation. In the event only 21 million doses were ready when mass inoculations started on 1 October. Legal liability was feared, especially as insurance companies refused cover. But Ford saw much merit in the program and doggedly pressed on.

On 11 October three elderly people died of heart attacks while receiving shots in the same clinic. Public response became cautious, so the President took his injection on national TV.

In mid November the first case of the neurological Guillain-Barre syndrome (GBS) occurred. Others followed, but the significance was questionable. However, by 9 December there had been 26 cases of GBS, including three deaths. It was getting troublesome. The rate was about four times greater in the vaccinated than unvaccinated, so the occurrence was hardly due to chance.

This was the last straw for the detractors. So, after much soul searching, on 16 December Dr Sencer recommended the suspension of the program. The whole fiasco came to an end that afternoon, 'in the interests of public safety'.

Since Fort Dix there had been three cases in the whole country, and those were on pig farms. As a pandemic it was a complete non event. Ultimately, neither epidemiologists nor politicians received any kudos, indeed Sencer was sacked.

Yet it was not just lack of cases which killed off the vaccination plan, but a mixture of the feared association of GBS (532 cases in the end), the problems of liability insurance allied with ill-understood informed consent and inadequate supplies.

During the 77 days of the loudly touted and politically expedient program, 44 million people were vaccinated. The other presidential candidate, Jimmy Carter, did not have a shot and went on to win the election; there must be a message in there somewhere.

(JL)

7
Disasters

Burke and Hare

From time to time medical schools ask for bodies for dissection. Nothing precipitous you understand; they do not want them until after the actual death of the owner. This requirement has not always been the case; in times past, some students got their material by other means.

In the time of Hippocrates, about 2,400 years ago, human dissection was expressly forbidden, in either the dead or the living. This restriction delayed advances in medical expertise for hundreds of years, until, in fact, AD 1540. That year, the Belgian anatomist Andreas Vesalius, then in his twenties, defied this ancient restricting convention and became the first to do the heretical deed whilst having in mind to further learning rather than to satisfy an idle curiosity.

In the very same year, Henry VIII allowed that surgeons were somehow more worthy than their then professional associates, barbers, and awarded them two executed criminals a year for dissection. A little niggardly for such sanguinary times, perhaps.

Subsequently the gallows were a rich source of raw material, and 200 years later they gave William Hunter the chance to set up his School of Anatomy in Great Windmill Street, London. Today, if you can drag yourself away from the strip shows down this side street off Shaftesbury Avenue, you will see a plaque commemorating the event (high on a wall of the Lyric Theatre on the corner of the two roads).

In Edinburgh the students, eager as ever, could sometimes be a little previous in getting the criminals off the gibbet. One poor unfortunate came round during an unseemly post-drop scramble. She lived on for years as Half-Hangit Maggie.

Having now arrived in Edinburgh, let's look at medicine's most famous accumulators of bodies. For it was there that the redoubtable William Burke and William Hare conducted their grisly and dubious business activities to provide bodies for the medical school.

In 1826 there succeeded to the Chair of Anatomy in Edinburgh an inspirational teacher, born orator and military surgeon veteran of Waterloo, Robert Knox. Such was his charisma that within a couple of years his class numbered over 500, comprising not just medical students but lawyers, artists and gentlemen with time on their hands. As all wanted a piece of the action, bodies came to be in short supply.

Knox loved his job, especially the adoration it generated, but he had a logistic problem: he needed the meat. So he enlisted the aid of several sportive students as well as a number of devious men-about-town to supply bodies, no questions asked.

On the night of 29 November 1827 two new suppliers brought Dr Knox an old man in a sack; he paid out £7 10s for the body. It should be stressed that the man was dead all right, and from natural causes. He had been, in fact, an army pensioner who had snuffed it at the lodging house of one of the vendors, William Hare. Hare owed his landlord £4 back rent, and fellow lodger William Burke had the sublime idea that cash may be turned over from this grave situation by selling to Knox.

It took only a moment to crack open the coffin, pop the corpse back in bed, fill the empty box with the appropriate weight in tanners bark, and then let the pitifully few mourners in to wring their hands and squeeze out the odd tear. Doubtless none keened with greater vigour or managed more snivels than Messrs Burke and Hare themselves.

Although to these two layabouts it may have seemed a mortal sin to let something rot underground when it could be sold for £7 10s on top of the ground, dead bodies were not in steady and guaranteed supply. They had a merchandise-flow problem, so they decided to create their own product.

The first to present was a miller who lived in the house. He was ill anyway, so no qualms were felt over his suffocation. £10 was the negotiated fee.

Next a passing beggarwoman was invited in, filled with whisky, strangled, nailed in a tea chest and delivered to the good doctor, who was delighted with the freshness of the goods.

The fee was the same for each, but, as with all businesses, there were expenses—alcohol and a box, for instance. So the carve-up of profits was less.

Two more unfortunates met similar fates. A prostitute, Mary Patterson, was met by Burke in a tavern, taken home to breakfast, filled with whisky, despatched before lunch and delivered in the afternoon. Her unforeseen appearance gave one of the students a nasty turn as he had known her professionally shortly before—in her profession, not his. This was young Fergusson, later to become Sir William Fergusson, Sergeant-Surgeon to Queen Victoria herself, no less. Doubtless he kept this bit of intelligence from her.

Burke became so bold he even relieved two policemen of a drunken woman on the pretext that he knew where she lived and would conduct her home. The lads were honing their arcane skill into an art form.

They had a rewarding day at the end of June 1828. An old lady and her grandson were dispatched, but on the way to Knox's establishment by horse-drawn cart, the animal collapsed between the shafts of its cart, so Burke and Hare collected from both the medical school and the knacker's yard.

In all, their stock in trade garnered between 15 and 32 unsuspecting and usually impoverished down-and-outs. The exact figure is unknown.

It came to an end after nine months, when two other lodgers at the infamous boarding house grassed on them. The police found the last of the macabre line in Dr Knox's cellar. Burke and Hare were arrested and charged with murder.

Their trial started at 10 a.m. on the morning of Christmas Eve 1828 and continued non-stop until 9.30 on Christmas morning, when Burke was found guilty. Hare, of course, would have suffered a similar fare had he not turned king's evidence and slipped through the system.

The judge had no hesitation in passing a sentence of death by hanging, his only agony was to decide whether Burke's body should hang in chains or his skeleton be preserved as a ghoulish warning to other like-minded villains. In the event, and fittingly, it was taken for dissection.

The execution itself was carried out publicly before a morbidly curious audience who were prepared to pay anything between five and 20 shillings for a window seat. Some 25,000 people attended what was obviously a gala event.

As the rope tightened, a shout went up for Knox to follow. He was a little hurt at the imprecations flung at him, considering it not to be within his academic duty to question the origins of still-warm specimens.

Knox himself appointed a committee of Scottish noblemen and gentry to examine his alleged connection. The committee's subsequent whitewash job buttered no parsnips as far as the canny citizens of Auld Reeky were concerned, and in 1840 he was forced to leave Edinburgh, together with fame and fortune. He went to London, studied the anatomy of whales and died in obscurity in 1862.

There were some sequels to the sordid episode. The government was compelled to regulate such matters as medical dissection by the passage of the Anatomy Act in 1832. Burke gained dubious posthumous glory by having his name pass into the language—'to burke', meaning to kill secretly by suffocation or strangulation, or to hush up.

Many years later a postscript to the story emerged. In 1986 Professor Matthew Kaufman was appointed to the Chair of Anatomy at Edinburgh and during his early explorations of the rambling department he came across a hitherto forgotten collection of about 300 plaster death masks They had been bought by the anatomy unit from the Edinburgh Phrenological Society (who else) over a hundred years previously and promptly forgotten.

Among them, besides the likeness of Mendelssohn, John Keats, Isaac Newton and Dr Samuel Johnson, was the cast of William Burke's head. Although he appears to have been somewhat out his league, he was probably better known to the public at large than any of the other artistic or intellectual giants in the collection.

(JL)

The blight of the Irish

Having watched their oats, turnips and wheat ... trampled, burned and raided by English armies, the peasants recognised the potato as a vegetable that could be cultivated and stored in secret ... that could endure the malevolence of the English (Andrew Nikiforuk)

The potato first came from the mountains of Bolivia and Peru, and fed the crews of Spanish ships returning to the Old World.

It is not known how the Irish first came across potatoes. Perhaps from hulks of Spanish ships washed onto their coast after the defeat of the Armada in 1588. Or perhaps Sir Walter Raleigh planted potatoes from Virginia on his Irish estates.

In any case, Irish peasants took up the new plant far more eagerly than other Europeans. It was to prove both a blessing and a curse to the Irish. By the 1590s, the potato was a key part of their diet.

No other crop grown on only one acre could feed a man, his wife and six children. For breakfast, lunch and dinner they had potatoes and milk. A working man would eat up to 6 kilograms of potatoes each day! Pigs, chickens, dairy cattle and family could all eat from the one cauldron.

Peasants banked and spent potatoes almost like money. They had many names for the potato: pratie, prata, fata, taters and Murphy. They even called themselves 'praties with a bone'. There were several warnings of the Great Famine. One came as early as 1740, when a bad frost killed most of the Irish crops. Starvation, typhus and dysentery ('fevers and fluxes') killed about 300,000.

But the ultimate tragedy came in 1845 after 17 shaky harvests, with various pests and diseases already affecting Ireland's potatoes.

According to J.S. Schapiro, 'The failure of the potato crop ... resulted in a great famine that brought the climax of suffering to a people already half starved.'

The potato blight travelled from the United States and came to Ireland via England. Eventually it hit all the potato-growing countries of Northern Europe.

The fungus had originally been a benign companion of the wild potato in the Andes. But the relationship went sour after the potato crossed the Atlantic. Several factors increased the ravages of the fungus and made this famine especially devastating.

July 1845 was unusually cold and rainy. Moreover, potatoes in Ireland were planted close together, as most farms were so small. So the spores could easily spread over what started as Ireland's largest-ever potato crop.

The first sign of blight was the stench. Affected plants blackened and withered in the ground; even those tubers which looked sound rotted once they were stored. As Nikiforuk says, 'the fungus ... sucked the life out of both the potato and its cultivator'.

Ironically, the potato itself had encouraged the population explosion which worsened the devastation of the blight.

It has been estimated that between 1760 and 1840 the population grew from 1.5 million to 9 million; a sixfold increase in just 80 years! Disraeli called Ireland the most densely populated country in Europe. The overpopulation was worst in the west. It was Oliver Cromwell who, two centuries before, had forced many Irish into the barren western province of Connaught.

The infestation killed over half the crop of 1845, wiped out that of the following year, and returned again in 1847 and 1848. Some historians believe the Famine continued until 1851.

Famine was also widespread elsewhere in Northern Europe, but because of their dependence on the potato, it hit the Irish hardest.

Among the deadly diseases were typhus ('black fever') and relapsing (yellow) fever, both transmitted by the common louse which flourished.

Whole families dragged themselves to cemeteries, dug their own graves and quietly lay down. Doctors and clergy did what they could; some of them died as well.

Some Englishmen said the famine reports were exaggerated. Subsidised imports of corn came late, and were then poorly distributed; many Irishwomen didn't know how to cook corn.

By 1847 (the third year of the Famine), the English Treasurer Charles Trevelyan organised soup kitchens for 3 million people.

According to Máire and Conor Cruise O'Brien:

Historians, both English and Irish, generally see the outbreak of famine as inevitable, but think that disaster on the scale which actually occurred could have been avoided by more determined governmental action ... Some individual Englishmen, and groups of Englishmen and Irishmen—notably the Society of Friends [Quakers]—did all that they could...but help on the great scale which alone would have sufficed to avert it was not forthcoming.

In desperation, many Irish emigrated. Yet, as Cecil Woodham-Smith says, 'they did not leave fever behind; fever went with them, and the path to a new life became a path of horror.'

It took emigrants about two months of further starvation and disease to cross the Atlantic to America in 'coffin ships'. These had too little food and water, were overcrowded and 'dangerously antique in construction", according to Woodham-Smith. Many captains buried half their passengers at sea.

In America, the survivors rented damp, dark one-room cellars for families of a dozen plus a pig or two. Other, even poorer Irish, sank into the ghettos of Liverpool, Manchester or Glasgow.

Yet others of course started afresh in Australia.

When the Famine struck, the population of Ireland was perhaps 9 million. By 1851, famine and fever claimed between half a million and 2 million. Another 1–2 million emigrated, or died in the attempt. Since those terrible times, the Irish have controlled their population, which is now only about half of that before the Famine.

Ireland commemorated the 150th anniversary of the Famine with the theme: 'Look back in sorrow, not in anger.'

(GB)

Typhoid Mary

It is 70 years since the death of Mary Mallon. 'Mary who?' you may well ask. Mary Mallon, who for years strode through New

York society like a grim reaper, dispensing typhoid bacteria with deadly and feckless abandon.

The word 'typhoid' is from the Greek *typhos*, meaning smoke or cloud, and refers to the floating confusion which occurs in the later stages of the malady. It is one of the so-called enteric fevers which cause gastroenteritis. The causative bacillus enters the body through contaminated food or water, and, once entrenched, there is an incubation period of seven to 14 days followed by malaise, loss of appetite and headache. At that stage it could be anything, but then a step like rise in temperature takes place to a hectic 104 degrees Fahrenheit (40 degrees Centigrade).

In the second week rose-coloured spots appear and later delirium. You then either recover very slowly or you die, and in inadequately treated cases, about nine per cent do just that.

Antibiotics are used now and are very effective. But in former days, about three per cent of sufferers who recovered remained long-term carriers, blissfully unaware they were shedding the bacteria from its hiding place in their gall bladder while at the same time suffering no ill effects themselves. If a carrier was a food handler and maintained poor hygiene, then he or she was a disaster waiting to happen. Such was Mary Mallon.

The typhoid bacillus has never been fussy where it gathered its prey, and has had some pretty up-market victims in its time. Prince Albert, consort of Queen Victoria, died of it, and their son, later to be Edward the VII, almost did. An earlier English king, Henry I, the 'Lion of England', succumbed, it was said, to the effects of a 'surfeit of lampreys', which was probably a euphemism for typhoid.

It caused almost 33 per cent of the deaths in the American Civil War, a conflict, incidentally, where another third died of other diseases, and only the remaining third of the deaths were in heroic circumstances. It was the cause of a major public health problem in the 1890s in Western Australia during the early rumbustious days of the discovery of gold in the

Coolgardie and Kalgoorlie area. Poor sanitation was the culprit in this instance.

Which brings us to the New York of 1900. In September that year a young man died of typhoid in the house in which Mary Mallon was staying. Nothing unusual about that; at the time such things were regarded as all part of life's immutable laws.

The next year she worked in a lawyer's house in Maine, and within a fortnight seven of the eight members of the household were down with the disease. Mary worked unstintingly in the sick-bay situation. So much so that she was given a $50 bonus. She and that outbreak were only connected years later. If she had but realised it then, of course, the tie up might have proved to have been a regular source of income for her—infect a family and then look after them.

Fairly frequently she moved from house to house in her job as a cook. For as Saki prophetically wrote at the time in another situation: 'The cook was a good cook, as cooks go. And as good cooks go, she went.'

She took a job in a Long Island house in 1909, whereupon six out of ten in the establishment promptly fell ill. Mind you, there were 3,467 cases in New York that year with 639 deaths, so at the time the disease was not regarded as the public-health scandal that it would be now. It was just the worm in the Big Apple, so to speak.

But on this occasion the medical fraternity did not sit around sucking their teeth or pursing their lips as they bemoaned the course of events whilst waiting to hit off on the second tee. No. A Dr George Soper went and smelt the drains and poked in the privy and pondered long and suspiciously over the local delicacy of giant clams. Disappointingly, none had been eaten.

'Well, has any other exotica been eaten, for goodness' sake?' wondered the exasperated doctor. The cook's tangy ice cream that had been everybody's favourite was a lame afterthought.

'Not the present cook, you understand, but the one who left three weeks ago just after the illness. Wait a minute, wait a minute. That's right, just after the typhoid started.'

Dr Soper took six harrowing months to track down Mary through a series of grief-stricken houses. In the end he knew she was a 40-year-old single woman and a migrant from Northern Ireland. Eventually, he ran her to ground in the kitchen of a top-drawer home in Park Avenue, New York.

One can picture the good doctor leaning slightly forward, placing the tips of his fingers together, and affecting his best bedside manner and wheedling tone, as he wondered aloud if she could see any possible connection between herself and the trail of people with hectic temperatures, rose-coloured spots and greenish diarrhoea who had remained behind as she had moved on, and who displayed all the characteristics of, er, um, typhoid.

Her answer was short, to the point and impressive: she attacked him with a meat cleaver.

He bolted, and so did she in the opposite direction—he to the police, she to the outside toilet.

In a new-found coyness for New York's finest, the sergeant shouted through the toilet door that he believed Miss Mallon could help with their enquires. Her answer was uncompromising, succinct and hurtful to any person's sensitivities about his or her parentage. So, with an inspector sitting on her chest, she was removed kicking and screaming and sent to the Riverside Hospital for communicable diseases.

There Dr Soper had her stools cultured, and it came as no surprise to anyone that they were teeming with typhoid bacilli. Again it fell to the lot of the luckless GP to explain to Mary that she was the carrier of a condition dangerous to other people, and that the germs were lodging in the stones in her gall bladder. Furthermore (and he must have braced himself as he told her this) the treatment was simple—have the gall bladder removed.

It is not necessary to draw pictures for you regarding her response. Suffice it to say that the interview room had prudently been stripped of potential missiles.

So she was kept incarcerated in the hospital for three years; brooding, malevolent, a study in suppressed anger. She worked in the laundry, retaining all the while those typhoid tombstones in her gall bladder, while at the same time honing to perfection a heart rending derring-do story for which her countryfolk are supposed to be famous. The upshot was that Mary Mallon was released after promising with all the vehemence she could muster, which was considerable, that she would stick to the copper rather than the casserole and report to the Health Department every three months.

She promptly disappeared, seemingly from the face of the earth. In fact she did what probably any upright, downright and forthright person would have done. She changed her name to Mrs Brown, and her job, surprise, surprise, back to cook.

For five more years Mary plied her deadly culinary art round New York city, while unsuspecting trenchermen wolfed her typhoid-ridden gobbets. In 1915 there was a serious outbreak in the Sloane Hospital for Women, where she was working. In a moment of ingenuous banter another cook called her Typhoid Mary, whereupon to everyone's surprise she fled. The police were notified and she was caught on Long Island. Rather disappointingly, she went like a lamb.

She was returned to the Riverside Hospital and given a life sentence of custodial care. By now the stuffing had been knocked out of her, even though the potent gall stones remained, and she went over to the enemy, so to speak, by becoming a worker in the hospital laboratory. The management even built her a small cottage in the grounds and she gave tea parties there. To accept an invitation no doubt meant playing rock-bun roulette, and perhaps was held as a kind of threat to the more obstructive patients.

Mary had a stroke in 1932 and died in 1938, not, as you may suppose, of the long-term complications of typhoid, but of bronchopneumonia. You will be relieved to know that she secreted the typhoid bacillus to the end.

When Mary Mallon died her score card was marked and the certainties came to ten outbreaks of typhoid fever which involved fifty-three cases and caused three deaths. Besides that she was almost certainly responsible for the 1904 outbreak at Ithaca in upstate New York when there were 1,400 cases. On top of these there were very many likely but unattributable episodes stretching back some thirty years.

Typhoid Mary touched scores of lives with her unique brand of ice cream; she terrorised dozens of policemen, insulted numerous public-health workers, and put the breeze up countless doctors. So spare her a passing thought as you abstractly drink your sparkling tap water, for it was by her polluting its likes that she accomplished much more in her lifetime than most of us are likely to do in ours.

(JL)

Painters dial R for death

Doctors learned about radium the same way they did about
X-rays: by trial and error (Catherine Caulfield)

In 1898 Marie and Pierre Curie announced their discovery of a new element. Radium fever swept the world.

In the United States, in 1915, Dr Sabin von Sochocky developed a luminous paint that he called 'Undark'. Next he founded the US Radium Corporation. His plant in New Jersey was only two blocks from Thomas Edison's laboratory, where Edison's assistant had received the radiation that later killed him. Should von Sochocky have read that as a warning?

US Radium's staff painted numerals onto watch dials and made crucifixes that glowed in the dark. The workers were women and girls, some only 12 years old. They used very fine brushes, which they brought to a point by pressing them between their lips. Sometimes, for fun, they painted their teeth or fingernails to glow in the dark.

In 1916 the medical journal *Radium* declared: 'Radium has absolutely no toxic effects, it being accepted as harmoniously by the human system as is sunlight by the plant.'

The First World War stimulated the demand for luminous dials on all sorts of instruments. By 1920, America had over 2,000 dial painters. But within four years, nine had died, reportedly of phosphorus poisoning, stomach ulcer, syphilis, anaemia, and cancer of the jaw. Many others had severe problems with their jaws and teeth.

Dr Theodore Blum, a dentist-doctor, reported a patient with an infected jaw 'caused by some radioactive substance used in the manufacturing, of luminous watch dials'.

In 1925 Dr Frederick Hoffman, statistician to Prudential Life Insurance, blamed radium poisoning. Working with him was Dr von Sochocky, who had resigned from his own company. By now, von Sochocky's own breath was more radioactive than that of his dial painters.

A team from the Harvard School of Public Health found the US Radium work area spattered with radium paint. In a dark room, the 'hair, faces, hands, arms, necks, dresses, underclothes ... of the dial painters were luminous', according to Caulfield.

All 22 workers tested had abnormal blood tests. The team concluded that all workers were exposed to excess radiation, both externally and internally. The deaths and illnesses, the Harvard team said, were 'due to radium'. The company threatened to sue if the team published its report.

Dr Harrison Martland, medical examiner for Essex County, home of US Radium, saw two dial painters with high radioactivity levels just before their deaths.

Researchers found that the optimists were wrong: radium does not pass straight through the body, but settles in bones, where it can cause cancer and damage the bone marrow.

Dial painters were not the only ones at risk.

Doctors were using radioactive substances for a hotchpotch of real and imaginary conditions: schizophrenia, rheumatism, high blood pressure, irregular periods, depression, poor sex drive and even debutante's fatigue!

In early 1925 US Radium's own chemist, Edwin Lehman, was well; within a month, he was dead of acute anaemia. Unlike the dial painters, he had not swallowed any paint, but had breathed in the radium.

Martland pressed for complete protective measures for workers using radioactive substances: in manufacturing plants, laboratories, hospitals and offices. But the lawyers still blamed poor hygiene and held up the publication of his report.

From 1925 on, the company was seldom out of the courts or the news.

In 1927 five former US Radium dial painters (the papers dubbed them 'The Five Women Doomed to Die') filed a case. Because workers' compensation in New Jersey did not cover radium poisoning, each woman sought damages of $250,000. One had endured 20 operations on her jaw, and had paralysed legs from spinal-cord damage. Two had to be carried into court; one could not even raise her hand to take the oath.

Defence lawyers invoked the two-year statute of limitations. Despite the media outcry, the court agreed; the women appealed. Legal wrangling held up the case for over a year, while the women faced painful deaths.

Well-wishers around the world sent prayers and advice. From France, Marie Curie suggested raw calf's liver. She herself was to die within a few years of radium-induced anaemia.

In May 1928, the women won permission to sue in the Supreme Court. But how long would that take? Suddenly a mediator appeared; within five days, he negotiated a settlement.

The company, 'Actuated solely by humanitarian considerations', gave each woman $10,000 and a yearly pension of $600, plus medical expenses.

Less than six months later, Dr Sabin von Sochocky himself died of aplastic anaemia. Radium had eaten away at his hands, mouth and jaw. Martland wrote: 'He ... gave all that was in him to help and comfort others suffering from this disease.'

It is sobering to consider that the painful deaths of these early victims led to safer working conditions for the makers of the atomic bomb, which in turn devastated the people of Hiroshima and Nagasaki.

(GB)

Wittenoom: the asbestos tragedy goes on and on

Peter Garrett and Midnight Oil have a song about it; Rolf Harris worked there. But it was Lang Hancock who, in the late 1930s launched blue asbestos mining at Wittenoom in the remote north of Western Australia.

Then the Second World War boosted world demand for this popular, versatile material; it could insulate pipes in submarines and filter noxious gases in gas masks.

In 1943 Hancock formed Australian Blue Asbestos Ltd, later bought out by CSR (Colonial Sugar Refineries).

Dr Eric Saint became Government Medical Officer for the whole of north-west Australia. Even from the air and 30 kilometres away, he could see the blue-grey asbestos dust over Wittenoom.

The offices alone had dust readings that would have been illegal down a mine. Thousands of tons of milling residue (tailings still containing asbestos) formed the roads and even coated the school playground. It was everywhere; dust levels were six to eight times the levels then considered 'safe'.

Inhaling asbestos particles causes asbestosis, a thickening or fibrosis of the lung tissue. In turn, this thickening blocks the flow of oxygen into the lungs and makes people breathless. One sufferer has compared it to 'having your lungs slowly filled with wet concrete'.

If asbestos levels are high enough, asbestosis may follow even fairly brief exposure, though it may not become apparent for many years after initial exposure. Malignant tumours that often follow asbestosis include lung cancer and mesothelioma.

Already workers were getting sick. From 1948 Dr Saint tried to convince the mine manager of the dangers, and then wrote to the Head of Public Health in Perth, predicting 'in a year or two, ABA will produce the richest and most lethal crop of asbestosis'.

Why did this message to the health department fall on deaf ears? Because some public servant wrote on the letter that Dr Saint was misinformed, and that no action was needed.

From 1959 Dr James McNulty was the local public health officer, but his best efforts were just as fruitless.

Only the Mines Department could order the company to clean up the mine, or close it down altogether. Dr McNulty kept warning the managers, and pressing his own chiefs, who in turn warned the Mines Department, but according to journalist and author Ben Hills, 'not a single prosecution was ever launched, no effective demands were ever made for safe ventilation ... the operation was never shut down for a single day'.

Dr McNulty's efforts with the men were just as frustrating:

'I must have told more than 100 of them: "you are sick, it is the asbestos, you must leave the mine". I don't think a single one of them ever took my advice.'

Residents accused him of destroying their town, and taking away their top incomes. The union wanted jobs at any price and pushed for an extra 20 cents an hour dust allowance!

In 1966 the Wittenoom mine and mill were shut down—not from guilt or remorse, but because the quarry was no longer economically viable. Not for another decade did the full health impact begin to emerge.

It was not only those in the mine or the mill who suffered. In 1950 Joan Joosten had moved to the nearby township of Wittenoom Gorge, as her husband was foreman at the mill. She worked as a secretary in the office; even there, dust hung in the air and clogged the flyscreens. The boss told Joan not to worry, as the dust was 'clean'. During her three years working for the mining company, she never had a chest X-ray.

Some 25 years later, Joan was getting tired, losing weight and had pains in the arms and chest; she had malignant mesothelioma. Joan battled her growth, and battled the company as well. Her husband sold his sandwich bar to look after her and pay legal costs.

But in 1979 Justice Wallace in the Supreme Court dismissed their case: 'I do not condemn as negligence that which, in my opinion, was a sad misadventure.'

This verdict seems to have overlooked all the evidence already available well before Joan came to Wittenoom in 1950. In 1931, Britain legislated to control dust levels in asbestos textile factories. In 1935, there were reports of lung cancer in patients with asbestosis.

The tragedy was quite predictable; the evidence was right there. Doctors knew the score; managers who cared to look knew the score. But the public took longer to find out.

Though Joan was going downhill, the Joostens appealed. In March 1980, a few hours before the hearing of the appeal, Joan died. Her memorial is the Joan Joosten Centre, headquarters of the Asbestos Diseases Society of Australia.

Sadly, Joan Joosten is one of many—even by 1978, some 40 people had died of diseases related to the asbestos mining at Wittenoom.

Rusting sheds now mark Wittenoom. In late 1996 about 30 people still lived in the township.

The story is far from over. New cases of malignant mesothelioma are expected to rise to a peak around the year 2010.

Of 6,912 former employees at Wittenoom, the number predicted to get asbestosis, mesothelioma or lung cancer is almost 2,000. Even children of Wittenoom workers have developed asbestos diseases.

As Ben Hills wrote, '[Wittenoom] will go down in the history of this poisoned planet alongside Chernobyl, Bhopal and Minamata.'

(GB)

Syphilis in Tuskegee, Alabama

On 19 May 1997 Bill Clinton, President of the United States, apologised to survivors of a racist medical experiment that began in 1932 and ran for 40 years.

In July 1972, some 25 years before Clinton's apology, the American media were enjoying an abundance of news, scandals and controversy.

After Senator Thomas Eagleton (running mate to George McGovern) revealed his past history of depression requiring hospital admissions and shock treatment, the public outcry forced him to withdraw as candidate for vice-president.

Officials of the US Public Health Service (PHS) welcomed the Eagleton controversy since it diverted heat from the medical scandal that broke on the very same day.

For 40 years from 1932, the PHS had been following, but not treating, 412 poor black sharecroppers who had advanced syphilis and who lived around the county seat of Tuskegee in Macon County, Alabama. According to James H. Jones, this was 'the longest nontherapeutic experiment on human beings in medical history'.

Why would reputable doctors take part in such an inhumane experiment?

Remarkably, there was a precedent. Between 1891 and 1910, doctors at the Oslo Clinic in Norway had followed, but not treated, several hundred people with syphilis. Their report appeared in a leading German journal in 1929.

One reason, though certainly no justification, for the American study was to confirm the common belief that syphilis in black people is very different from syphilis in whites.

The Alabama subjects were not only black and poor; most were also illiterate. The PHS doctors, who were mostly white, had offered them free check-ups, free treatment for minor ailments, hot meals on clinic days, and burial stipends for their survivors.

When pressed by the media, PHS officials couldn't even find an experimental protocol. The experiment had just grown; it had included regular examinations, blood tests and above all, autopsies.

Dr J. Williams served as an intern at Andrews Hospital in Alabama's Tuskegee Institute. He said that despite official assurances about informed consent: 'The people … were not told what was being done.'

A survivor, Charles Pollard, said: 'They come around from time to time and check me over and they say: "Charlie, you've got bad blood" … they never mentioned syphilis to me.'

Worst of all, the men believed that PHS doctors were treating them for their 'bad blood'. An official letter offered 'your last chance to get a second examination … and after it … you will be given a special treatment'.

This was not treatment at all; it was a lumbar puncture (needle in the back to draw a sample of cerebrospinal fluid for testing). But to convince the men that this was treatment, the doctors called it a 'spinal shot'. Most men had side-effects from their lumbar puncture; over 40 years later, one said: 'I never have got over that shit.'

Dr Reginald James—who was not involved with the experiments—worked in Macon County from 1939 to 1941. When he found a man with syphilis, Eunice Rivers, the black nurse who kept track of the men, would warn him off: 'He's under experiment and not to be treated.'

If Dr James insisted on treating such patients, they never returned, since they knew they would lose their benefits. Moreover, they believed they were already having full treatment.

Belonging to 'Miss Rivers' Lodge' made them feel special.

How could they know that they were pawns in a deadly experiment?

PHS spokesmen defended themselves by pointing out that the experiment had been the subject of many medical conferences and journal articles. How could 100,000 medical readers fail to ask questions?

Moreover, PHS doctors convinced their private colleagues not to treat the experimental subjects for their syphilis. Instead, as the men fell ill, their doctors should just refer them to the hospital to ensure that they came to autopsy. Undeterred by blindness, paralysis, dementia and early death in some of their patients, the private doctors readily agreed to all this.

Once the story broke, *The Atlanta Constitution* newspaper condemned the 'moral astigmatism that saw these black sufferers simply as subjects in an experiment, not as human beings'.

One citizen called the experiment 'but another act of genocide by whites ... that again exposed the nature of whitey: a savage barbarian and a devil'.

Another asked: 'How in the name of God can we look others in the eye and say "This is a decent country"?'

Though he worked for the VD division of the Atlanta Centre for Disease Control, Dr Donald Printz said: 'A literal death sentence was passed on some of those people.'

But Dr John Heller, who had directed the VD division between 1943 and 1948, bluntly told reporters there had been nothing unethical or unscientific.

Some other doctors were just as blind. Dr R.H. Kampmeir of the Vanderbilt University admitted that many patients with syphilis would die if not treated: 'This is not surprising. No one has ever implied that syphilis is a benign infection.'

Apologists claimed that, in 1932, the available treatments (mercury, arsenic and bismuth) were worse than the disease. They said the drugs were painful, slow to act, toxic, and sometimes even fatal.

But no possible rationalisation could justify withholding penicillin after 1943 when it proved to be effective for syphilis.

Public pressure led to an independent inquiry. A panel of nine (of whom five were black) damned the experiment as 'ethically unjustified [even] in 1932'.

Senator Edward Kennedy held hearings on human experimentation. Two survivors, Charles Pollard and Lester Scott, told their story of illiterate blacks trusting the educated whites who had betrayed them. Each had been told that his blood was bad; each had gone along for 40 years with doctors who said they were treating him.

Outraged citizens of Tuskegee elected their first black mayor. Legislators passed tough regulations to protect subjects of medical experiments.

Over a century ago, Boston physician Dr Oliver Wendell Holmes noted: 'Medicine, professedly founded on observation, is as sensitive to outside influence, political, religious, philosophical, imaginative, as is the barometer to the atmospheric density.'

Even today, the Tuskegee study should sound a warning to researchers who argue against the need for ethics committees to oversee medical research.

(GB)

8

Addictions and Obsessions

That drowsy numbness: opium and the poets

Reports in the medical Press of the effects of hallucinogenic drugs on imagery and the spatial experience began early this century. But descriptions of similar blowouts had been part of literature long before that.

It is no secret that opium, usually taken as laudanum, affected the writings of such luminaries as Samuel Taylor Coleridge, George Crabbe, Francis Thompson, even the sublime John Keats himself. Thomas De Quincey's well-known narrative on the narcotic experience is brazenly entitled *Confessions of an English Opium-eater* (1822), and in it he describes its pleasures thus: 'Thou hast the keys of Paradise, oh just, subtle, and mighty opium.' Mind you, he also damns the pain as 'An Iliad of woes'.

Coleridge (1772–1834) is perhaps the best-known opium taker in this medley, and apparently it gave him the impetus to write his famous 'Kubla Khan'. The story goes that during a drug-induced sleep the author imagined life's impenetrable secret had been revealed to him. He woke, feverishly began to set it all down, was interrupted by an inopportune visitor, and never recaptured the mood when he departed. Nonetheless his last lines are significant:

Weave a circle round them thrice,
And close your eyes with holy dread:
For he on honey dew hath fed,
And drunk the milk of paradise.

Keats, Crabbe and Thompson were all medically trained, and their recreational use of opiates is revealed in some of their verses, though none attempts an objective account of the definitive drug experience.

Clinically, hallucinations vary with dosage and frequency of use. The most common is a distortion of space and time in which both can seemingly expand to infinity. Visual hallucinations are more common than auditory and olfactory ones, and can range from bright lights to bizarre but recognisable images. A sense of depersonalisation and terror can be identified in several poems. All in all, true addiction is more often seen in poorly socialised and dependent personalities than in well-structured ones, and in poets no less than in anyone else.

George Crabbe (1754–1832) became a surgeon apothecary after apprenticeship in the country. Travel to London to pursue a literary career was the preferred choice, but eventually he became a parson. He began taking opium in 1790 after having been given it for vertigo, and continued to imbibe it daily for the remaining 42 years of his life. The resulting delusions were mainly concerned with terror and pursuit. Crabbe's most famous literary work is *The Borough*, on which Benjamin Britten's 20th-century opera *Peter Grimes* was based.

Francis Thompson (1859–1907) was first given laudanum on prescription for 'lung fever' while a medical student at Manchester. He was a somewhat withdrawn and unstable person, and became habituated for the last 27 years of his life. He came from Preston, a cotton-spinning town in darkest Lancashire, seemingly a most unlikely place for a sensitive poet to emerge. Anyway, Thompson never enjoyed studying medicine, failed continually for as long as his doctor father would support him, until after six meaningless years he took himself off, together with a goodly supply of laudanum, to London. There he lived as a derelict, moving between monasteries, writing of his drug-induced fantasies until he died, not of opium poisoning but tuberculosis.

His terrifying dreams he described as 'in part the worst realities of my life'. He wrote one poem which with touching frankness he called 'The Poppy'. It is full of narcotic-induced fantasies where the poppy emerges as 'the withered flower of dreams'.

Of all the English poets who dabbled in drugs his was the talent it most profoundly affected, reaching its apotheosis in *The Hound of Heaven*, where, in his mind, he is pursued by God:

> I fled Him down the night and down the days;
> I fled Him down the arches of the years;
> I fled Him down the labyrinthine ways
> Of my own mind.

In Thompson's evocative piece 'At Lords', he describes a visit to watch his old county, Lancashire, play Middlesex at cricket at Lords. It finishes with these famous lines, which, notwithstanding the inferred symbolism, are very moving:

> The field is full of shades as I near the shadowy coast,
> And the ghostly batsman plays the bowling of a ghost,
> And I look through my tears on the soundless-clapping host
> As the run-stealers flicker too and fro,
> Too and fro:
> O my Horn by and my Barlow long ago!

John Keats (1795–1824), the son of a livery-stable keeper, was an occasional laudanum taker, not an addict. He was apprenticed to a surgeon in Edmonton, Middlesex, but moved to

Guy's Hospital where he qualified as an apothecary in 1816. He abandoned medicine for literature after six months.

In 1819 he was hit in the eye by a cricket ball, and his house-mate, Charles Brown, wrote that he received opium after this event, as he had done on occasions before. The poet, though never admitting to taking the poppy, wrote the next day how he had slept in, felt languid, and was indifferent to pain and pleasure.

If any of Keats's poems imply the effect of opium, it is his 'Ode to the Nightingale'. It was written within six weeks of the cricket-ball incident, and the first few lines are pretty explicit:

> My head aches and a drowsy numbness pains
> My senses, as though of hemlock I had drunk,
> Or emptied some dull opiate to the drains
> One minute past, and Lethe-wards had sunk.

In a trance-like state he hears the nightingale—possibly an auditory hallucination and later pleads for escape:

> Fade far away, dissolve and quite forget.

Later Keats has thoughts of death:

> Now more than ever seems it rich to die,
> To cease upon the midnight with no pain.

And he concludes, as though rousing from an opium-induced sleep, confused over reality:

> Was it a vision or a waking dream?
> Fled is that music: Do I wake or sleep?

William S. Burroughs, 20th-century author (*The Naked Lunch*) and self-confessed drug taker, has said that drugs heighten the awareness and imagination of a writer. Yet it seems to be a constant grievance of those who take hallucinogenic drugs that it is impossible to communicate in words the transcendental effects they produce. The great poets probably got nearer than anyone.

(JL)

Sigmund Freud and cocaine

It makes you hyper and smarter, faster and better…you know, sort of like the Six Million Dollar Man (25-year-old male, in Dan Waldorf's *Cocaine Changes*)

In 1860 the German pharmacologist Albert Niemann isolated cocaine, one of the ingredients in the leaves of the South American coca plant. He wrote that it leaves 'a peculiar numbness, followed by a sense of cold when applied to the tongue'.

Despite this observation, Niemann overlooked cocaine's potential as a local anaesthetic. Only a few years later, a French pharmacologist did suggest that cocaine might be a useful local anaesthetic. But he did not follow it up either.

One of the first doctors to experiment with cocaine on humans was Dr Sigmund Freud. In 1884 he was only 28, a poor, little-known but ambitious doctor at the famous General Hospital in Vienna, when he wrote a letter to his fiancée Martha Bernays in which he enthused about cocaine, 'which some Indian tribes chew to make themselves resistant to privation and fatigue'.

Freud ordered one gram of cocaine, but was outraged to be charged about ten times the expected price. But before sending the cocaine straight back, he took one-twentieth of a gram. After a few moments, all his anger evaporated and he felt dramatically brighter: 'nothing at all one need worry about'.

One month later, Freud noted: 'I take small amounts regularly against depression and indigestion and with the most brilliant results.' He sent Martha cocaine to 'make her strong and give her cheeks a rosy colour'.

Soon Freud was mailing cocaine to relatives, sharing it with colleagues, and prescribing it for digestive disorders, weight loss and asthma, for morphine and alcohol addiction, and even as an aphrodisiac. Just on the strength of 'some dozen experiments', he wrote an enthusiastic paper.

His biographer Dr Ernest Jones called him a 'public menace' on cocaine.

One of Freud's friends, Dr Fleischl, had become a morphine addict. American doctors were treating morphine addicts with cocaine, and Freud did the same for his friend. Fleischl did well at first.

Another friend, Dr Carl Koller, was searching for an effective local anaesthetic for eye surgery. He wrote about a colleague who 'partook of some cocaine with me from the point of a penknife and remarked 'How that numbs the tongue.' The observation was not new, but it was Koller who took it further.

Would cocaine numb the eye as it numbed the tongue?

> We [Koller and Freud] trickled the cocaine solution under the upraised lids of each other's eyes. Then we put a mirror before us, took a pin in hand and tried to touch the cornea with its head … We could make a dent in the cornea without the slightest awareness of the touch …

Soon Koller presented his findings to the Viennese Medical Association. As the news spread, wags called Dr Carl Koller 'Coca Koller'.

Freud's own father was one of the first patients to enjoy a painless operation for glaucoma, with Koller and Freud giving a local anaesthetic of cocaine. An American cavalry officer even wanted Koller to sail for the United States and examine his horse!

William Martindale, future president of the Pharmaceutical Society of Great Britain, advised the English to give up tea and take coca instead.

But by July 1885, Freud's addicted friend Dr Fleischl was taking a full gram of cocaine each day. Worse, he had convulsions and hallucinations of white snakes. Freud sometimes sat up all night with his friend.

The man who had hoped to become the first European to be cured of morphine addiction by cocaine was now the first European cocaine addict.

Freud may have believed that cocaine was not addictive because it did not produce the dramatic withdrawal crisis of opium or morphine. One critic called cocaine 'the third scourge of mankind'. The fiasco shattered Freud's early reputation. But he reportedly continued not only to use, but also to prescribe cocaine until at least 1895.

Was Freud just unlucky in this early cocaine phase of his career? Had he, like Koller, concentrated on its anaesthetic effects, would he have become a famous anaesthetist instead of the father of psychoanalysis?

In his last paper on cocaine, Freud finally admitted that it did harm morphine addicts and produce:

> ... physical and moral deterioration, hallucinatory states of agitation similar to delirium tremens, a chronic persecution mania ... hallucinations of small animals moving in the skin and cocaine addiction instead of morphine addiction.

Four years after Fleischl's death, Freud was still blaming himself: 'I had been the first to recommend the use of cocaine ... The misuse of that drug ... hastened the death of a good friend'.

But later, Freud omitted references to some of his early papers promoting cocaine. Was this deliberate? Did he just happen to forget? Or was the great Freud himself subject to Freudian slips?

(GB)

Percy Grainger's and William Gladstone's curious obsession

The death in 1994 of a British politician who was found dressed in women's stockings, and who had suffocated while allegedly engaging in some sort of solitary sexual burlesque brought attention to such goings on, especially when they involved prominent people. Such activities are almost certainly not as uncommon as we may think.

Percy Grainger was born in Melbourne in 1882, and showed exceptional musical talent from early childhood. He became one of the foremost pianists of this century and probably Australia's most highly regarded composer ('Handel in the Strand', 'Country Gardens', etc.). On top of this he at once led an eccentric private existence and extroverted public life.

Grainger's father, John, was an architect, but also an alcoholic and syphilitic. Percy himself did not have the disease, but his mother, Rose, did. Although she doted on the talented boy, Rose feared he would follow his father's decline, so she horsewhipped him when he showed signs of straying from his piano practice.

Out of this there developed a most unusual relationship of mutual dependency between mother and son. She managed both his professional and private life, and though an incestuous relationship has been speculated upon, the many letters each left seem to exclude this. Suffering from neurosyphilis, Mrs Grainger committed suicide in 1922.

The harsh discipline and perverse ambience of his childhood, buoyed by a fancy for literature associated with cruelty, had directed Percy's sexual urges along an abnormal path: sadomasochism. From the age of 16, 'wildness, recklessness and unbridled savagery were the keynotes of his existence … guilt and shame had little place in his life' as his biographer John Bird puts it.

So diligent was he in beating himself—or getting others to do so—that blood usually flowed, and he laundered his own shirts to conceal the evidence. Girlfriends were drawn into these activities, and pleasure heightened by recording the excesses on film. As mute testimony, he would hold up to the camera a notice with details of the kind of whip used, number of lashes as well as type of film and exposure on which it had been recorded!

In 1928 Grainger married Ella Strom, a Swedish artist and poet, the ceremony taking place at the Hollywood Bowl. Ella was under the impression that this was a kind of secluded glade and was astounded to find herself taking the vows in front of 28,000 people to the accompaniment of a 126-strong choir and orchestra performing her husband's new piece, 'To A Nordic Princess'. That's style for you.

The beatings continued, and shared sessions with his wife became so violent the musician felt it prudent to deposit a letter indicating that should death in either follow a bout of flogging, that, in fact, to him flagellation was the highest manifestation of love.

Both survived the onslaught, however, and Percy died of carcinoma of the prostate at the age of 78.

Quite apart from all this self-inflicted brutality, Percy Grainger showed a remarkable lack of proportion, an exaggerated emotionalism and a flamboyant eccentricity. He bequeathed his skeleton to the Percy Grainger Museum 'for preservation and possible display'. Some of his whips are also in the museum's collection.

Such characteristics were quite unlike those displayed by our second flagellating VIP. Indeed, this second man was looked upon as the very model of Victorian virtue, piety and rectitude.

He was William Ewart Gladstone, four times British prime minister, over 60 years in Parliament, unexcelled at verbal reticulation and master of the subordinate clause.

In 1839, at the age of 29, Gladstone married Catherine Glynne. She was to bear him eight children and provide him with a secure home base. It was said she was a woman of wit, charm and complete discretion, which is just as well for all his life Gladstone kept a diary in which he wrote about 'wounds from his secret conflict'.

In 1843, at the age of 34, he speculated in his diary as to 'how far satisfaction ... delighting in pain may be a true phenomena of the human mind'. And then on 13 January 1849 he confided, 'having been much tempted ... I made a slight application of a new form of discipline ... how thankful ought I to be if I should find it to so continue'.

Regrettably for him, gratification declined and he confessed it was becoming a convenient cover for 'unabated impurity'. He tentatively recommended to himself, via the diary, that rescue work among prostitutes may lift the effect.

So Gladstone became a member of an Anglo-Catholic group which did a variety of 'good works' among the underprivileged; the saving of 'fallen women' he saw as his contribution.

Thus in 1851 he got out into the world of the demimonde, where, incredibly, he distributed copies of *Uncle Tom's Cabin* as a suitably uplifting tract. Whether he partook of these women's professional charms is not certain, and vehemently denied later by his children, but in July he noted he 'trod the path of danger'.

His thoughts not being always altruistic, he felt shame at their sexual content, a feeling he gratifyingly found best overcome by self-flagellation. Flogging sessions would be indicated in the diary not by a word, but a drawing of a whip.

Gladstone particularly sought the company of a young woman called Elizabeth Collins, and she is written up many times with tantalising vagueness. For instance, on 13 July 1851 he enigmatically wrote of a two-hour 'strange and humbling scene'. Naturally, it led to the scourge.

To the statesman, Elizabeth was 'lovely beyond measure'. Indeed, her attractions were enough to make him take early leave of a dinner given by Lord Palmerston in order to spend two hours with her; to be followed, of course, by the chastening whip. I wonder what Palmerston and his guests would have made of it if they had known.

Gladstone was both smitten and unnerved by Miss Collins, and after 17 meetings of mixing 'impurity' and 'rescue', he wondered if it were not unlawful. It took an unconscionable time for the politician to make up his mind and he confided to his diary that, paradoxically, the beatings were as much an encouragement as a deterrent for impure temptation. For a man in his position the moral conflict must have been considerable. Nevertheless, when dear Miss Collins migrated to Australia the chance to stop was allowed to slip and she was replaced by others.

Twice at least he was recognised. With one, blackmail was threatened. Gladstone, fearing for his public credibility, sued, won, and the blackmailer got 12 months' hard labour!

The other was even more embarrassing. A well-intentioned but unthinking observer sent a letter to the *Times*, no less, saying he had seen an elderly man annoying two ladies, but as he recognised the gent to be Gladstone, realised he must have been acting with the 'highest honour'!

If those in the public eye find gratification in behaviour which is liable to outrage middle-class morality, better they keep it under wraps; contemporary attitudes may prove to be less tolerant than was the case with W.E. Gladstone or G.P. Grainger.

(JL)

9
Longevity

The oldest of the old

In January 1995 Lady Elliot of Harewood died in England at the age of 90. Not a stupendous age nowadays, but two facets of her life made her remarkable. First, she was the first woman—apart from a queen—ever to speak in the House of Lords. Second, and more interestingly as a contributor to medical history, her father was born as long-ago as 1823, when Napoleon was only two years dead and Beethoven finally became stone deaf. More than that, her grandfather was born in 1768, at the beginning of the Industrial Revolution and while Dr Johnson and Mozart were in full flight. So, incredibly, it took 227 years to complete three generations.

The 'oldest of the old' are a fascinating group of people; they are vintage models representing the most indestructible members of society. Mind you, in times past, ages were often exaggerated due to lack of records or poor memory or financial gain.

For instance, Thomas Parr was reputed to have been 152 when he died in 1635. Despite any doubts which may have been harboured, in his dotage he was well regarded enough to have his portrait painted and later hung in the then new

Ashmolean Museum in Oxford. It is still there over 300 years on. William Harvey examined the body but wisely made no comment on the age.

Englishman Thomas Cam was born in 1471 and was said to have lived through 10 complete reigns until he died aged 207. Actually, on careful examination, the figure 2 has been superimposed over 1 on his tombstone.

It was not until the 1830s that the recording of dates of births became compulsory in Western countries and we got some order into things.

According to the *Guinness Book of Records* (1994 edition), the oldest person authentically recorded in Australia was Caroline Maud Mockridge. She was born on 11 December 1874 and died aged 112 years 330 days on 8 November 1987. In 1992 there were about 1,500 centenarians in Australia.

For years it was claimed that the oldest person ever to have survived with provable dates was a man from a remote Japanese island. Born in 1865, he died in 1986 aged 120 years and 237 days. He worked on the farm until he was 105, took up smoking at the age of 70 and attributed his long life to 'God, Buddha and the Sun' (not smoking, thank goodness). But even this great age has been superseded by a grand old lady, Jeanne Calment. She lived in Arles, France, and was born in 1875. As a girl she met Vincent Van Gogh, whom she described as 'scruffy'. She died in 1997 aged 122.

Famous people who have cracked the 100 are Grandma Moses, the 'Primitive Painter' from America, who died aged 101, and Irving Berlin, the composer, also 101 at the end. Comedian George Burns at 97 said he could not die—he's booked. He eventually succumbed in 1996 at the age of 100 years and two months.

The last surviving soldier of the American Civil War died in 1959, 94 years after it had finished.

According to the *Weekly Telegraph* of February 1994, the oldest working man in Britain was a 94-year-old motorcycle repair man in Birmingham who planned to ride his bike to see the Queen on his 100th birthday.

The 20th century has seen a dramatic increase in Western average life expectancy, from about 47 in 1900 to about 74.5 in males and 80 in females in the late 1990s. It has been postulated that if the body could retain its teenage physiology we could live for about 700 years. Though there are grounds for believing there is a finite lifespan, it may be longer than currently thought.

Though improving health status and independence are allowing more people to survive into very old age (over 85), there are no signs yet of any extension of the upper limit of human life. Between 1981 and 1991 the number of centenarians in the UK doubled, a trend projected to accelerate. In 1992 there were about 40,000 centenarians recorded worldwide, only 22 per cent of whom were men. It may be women encounter fewer hazards, such as war, work accidents, smoking and heart disease. Further, perinatal and some bacterial-caused mortality is greater in the male; perhaps the immune response is different in each.

Genetic influences, immune response, stress levels and environmental aspects contribute to the prolongation of life. All are factors which could account for the disproportionate number of grand seniors in three unique areas of the world.

Abkhazia, Georgia, in southern Russia between the Black and Caspian seas has always been on the crossroads of history and is well known for its centenarians. By contrast, Hunza, between Kashmir and Afghanistan, and Vilcabamba, Ecuador, in the Andean foothills breed their champions in remote splendour.

Documentation is rare, so years are estimated by major events—marriage, war service, heavy winters and so on. Correlating all factors, researchers have found discrepancies. For instance, a father's age may have been used to avoid military service and then retained.

Nonetheless, old age is a proved and common characteristic of the areas, and to the accepted theories have been added: pace of life (compare the giant tortoise with an average age of 120), physical activity, diet, and lack of self-abuse with drugs including nicotine, alcohol and the like. What has never been found is a fountain of magical spring water.

The longest living things of all are, of course, trees, the leader being a Bristlecone pine in Nevada at a verified 4,900 years.

Fascinating stories of distant personal contacts occasionally occupy the correspondence columns of the *Times*. Each tries to outdo the others. My only claim is that as a boy I (JL) met a man who had sat through the whole of the first ever Test Match in 1877! Or so he said.

Perhaps author Antonia Fraser has the best story. She recounts how as a child in Oxford in the 1930s she had met people who had known Dr Martin Routh of Magdalen College. He died in 1854 aged 99, and claimed that when young he had known an old lady who as a girl had seen Charles II walking his spaniels. As Charles died in 1685, this time stretch vies with that of Lady Elliot; perhaps akin to the tenuous contact in the song 'I danced with a man who danced with a girl who danced with the Prince of Wales'.

Can anyone challenge it?

(JL)

Alchemy, body-freezing or virgin's blood?

It's not the men in my life that counts—it's the life in my men
(Mae West)

Have you heard of the man whose lifelong ambition was to live to be 90 and then be shot dead by a jealous husband?

Alchemy, body-freezing, virgin's blood and snake venom are just a few of the devices we have used in our quest for a vigorous long life.

Movie actor George Burns's formula was optimism: 'With a little luck, there's no reason why you can't live to be 100.

Then you've got it made, because very few people die over 100.' And of course, Burns did make 100. Englishwoman Edith Beck would have made a good match for George Burns; on her 103rd birthday, she decided to look after her health and give up smoking. At 117, Leliai Omar Bin Datuk Panglima of Malaysia cycled 43 kilometres to marry his 40-year-old fiancée (his 18th wife)!

Many cultures hold that humans were once immortal. Tithonus, the Trojan, loved Eos, the goddess of dawn. She persuaded Zeus to make Tithonus immortal, but forgot to ask for his eternal youth. In the end, poor old Tithonus could only sit babbling in a locked room, so she changed him into a grasshopper.

Elixirs of life are prominent in Hindu, Hebrew, Arab and Greek cultures.

Over the centuries, many alchemists have been loonies, charlatans and plain quacks, but alchemy has also attracted respectable scientists like Isaac Newton. Alchemists pursued two main goals: to turn base metals into gold, and to produce an Elixir of Life.

In the 1st century BC, a Chinese alchemist advised his emperor to transmute mercury into gold, turn it into cutlery, eat with it, and so become immortal. Nothing to it!

The unconventional Swiss physician-alchemist Paracelsus (1493–1541) claimed to have distilled a potion of immortality from mercury.

The Italian adventurer who called himself Count Alessandro di Cagliostro (1743–1795) was short, fat, ugly, unwashed, rude and boastful. But he toured Europe in great style as an alchemist, flogging two famous elixirs. The first merely stopped a man from aging further, but the second rejuvenated him by ten, twenty or even thirty years. The proof? Cagliostro himself. He was thousands of years old, and remembered everything: the building of the Pyramids, the Roman emperors—history's greatest name-dropper!

The first elixir was blood. Romans drank the blood of slain gladiators. Some despots killed young virgins so they could drink or bathe in their blood, while others merely sucked their milk or inhaled their breath. Consider also the Christian practice of Holy Communion, in which wine representing the blood of Jesus is drunk: 'Whoso ... drinketh my blood, hath eternal life' (John 6:54).

Tribes in India reportedly lived 400 years by eating snakes. Prescriptions included an ounce of snake's urine, taken every morning for 15 days, every year, especially in spring. Snakes moulting were thought to be rejuvenating themselves. Hence, snakeflesh would rejuvenate humans, as would chickens fed on minced snake and even eggs laid by snake-fed birds.

In 1492, a Jewish physician transfused Pope Innocent VIII with the blood of several young men who then quickly died. When the pope died as well, the doctor had to make himself scarce.

One recipe for a long and healthy life is to eat less. This is not a new idea. Ecclesiasticus (37:24) warns us about overeating: 'By surfeiting many have perished: but he that is temperate, shall prolong life.'

The Venetian nobleman Luigi Cornaro confessed in his *Discourses on the Sober Life* (1558) that riotous living had left him at the age of 45 with gout, fever and stomach pains. His doctors gave him up, but he became a model of temperance and lived to 103.

The German physician Christoph Hufeland (1762–1836) wrote lifestyle and diet recipes that anticipated modern diets, not only in content, but also in the title: *Makrobiotik*.

The message today is similar: eat less, but have enough fibre, protein, fat, vitamins and minerals. Animal experiments show that this actually works.

Dairy farmers should forever toast the Russian Nobel Prize winner of 1908, microbiologist Ilya Metchnikoff (1845–1916).

He attributed ageing largely to a 'putrefying bowel' (slow poisoning by toxins produced by bowel bacteria). Among his fans was Louis Armstrong, who took nightly laxatives and lived to the age of 71, and Mae West, who was hooked on daily enemas and lived to 87.

Metchnikoff attributed the longevity of Bulgarians partly to their yoghurt, in which he found bacteria that eliminated the noxious bacteria in the bowel. In his lab, Metchnikoff kept a large pot of Bulgarian yoghurt, which he offered to all visitors. To this day, New Zealand makes Metchnikoff yoghurt with natural acidophilus and bifidus 'to aid digestion'.

Another popular way to keep down the nasty bugs in your bowel was to have part of it surgically removed.

In the 1920s Dr John Brinkley of Kansas ran his own radio station KFKB ('Kansas First, Kansas Best'). Between fundamentalist sermons and country music, he talked into his gold-plated microphone and promoted his method of rejuvenation: transplanting slices of goat testicles into grateful old men. Before losing his licence in 1929, he earned over US$1 million a year and was able to lend one of his three yachts to the Duke and Duchess of Windsor. By contrast, Henry Leighton Jones (1868–1943) of Morisset, New South Wales, who transplanted monkey glands in the 1930s, was a reputable mainstream GP.

Swiss physician Paul Niehans injected cells from unborn lambs into Konrad Adenauer, Winston Churchill, Pope Pius XII and Charlie Chaplin. Dr Ana Aslan spent years promoting Gerovital, which contained novocaine (a local anaesthetic) plus a secret ingredient. During the 1950s she treated over 5,000 elderly patients, including Somerset Maugham, Charles de Gaulle, and Konrad Adenauer (who tried everything, but died in 1967 at the age of 81 nonetheless).

Some optimists have frozen themselves into suspended animation and waited for medical miracles to revive them.

This freeze-thaw technique (cryonics) started with physicist Robert Ettinger in the 1950s. Even now, the faithful lie patiently frozen in cryonics centres all over world.

One of the cyronics centres, the Alcor Life Extension Foundation in California, hit the headlines in 1988. Inside a vat of liquid nitrogen somebody found the frozen bodyless head of Dora Kent, mother of cryonics guru Saul Kent. Allegedly, Kent had first transferred her from a convalescent home as she was near death (then 83), then had her decapitated and frozen without medical help. But was she alive before she lost her head? The police found four more frozen heads and a frozen body; the lawyers had a ball.

There is an even simpler approach to death—denial. Columnist Peter Smark wrote in the *Sydney Morning Herald* of 15 November 1997: 'The American middle class, for instance, firmly believes that death is optional. So when a member of the group dies, it is his or her own fault. Or a doctor's. Or an accountant's. A lawsuit often results.'

There are three regions in the world—Abkhazia, Hunza and Vilcabamba—in which we still hear of active, healthy people living to even 150. We can speculate about these pockets of longevity. Is it their active lifestyles, freedom from stress or sparse diets? Or is it merely their poor record-keeping and illiteracy? Whereas trees have rings and fish have scales, there are no accurate markers of human age.

The consensus view doubts whether people have actually lived beyond 110 or 120 years. Most of us will not get as far as that: our own biological clocks make it unlikely that we will match George Burns and reach 100.

The *maximum* lifespan has probably not increased greatly over the centuries. What has changed is the *average* life expectancy at birth.

There's a definite gender difference in longevity: 78 per cent of the world's recorded centenarians are female. Moreover, spinsters outlive married women, whereas married men outlive bachelors. All this reinforces the feminist messages: women are stronger, and marriage is great for guys, but woeful for women.

If you're looking for longevity, choose the right ancestors. To estimate your life expectancy, take the average years of life of your parents and all four grandparents.

But don't stop there: improve your odds by working on your lifestyle and risk factors.

Some enthusiasts recommend taking melatonin, while others pin their hopes on DHEA (de-hydro-epi-androsterone).

Travel can work wonders too. Japan has bathhouses with solid-gold tubs. True believers pay heaps to soak there. Don't laugh—the Japanese live longer than people of any other country.

(GB)

A Final Word: Can Immunisation Alone Save Third World Children?

Fog had delayed the tiny plane; everyone in the tiny mountain village high in the Andes was still waiting. Then a message came. the pilot would have to come after dark.

Children ran all around the village, calling out: 'The pilot is coming; come and bring a torch for him.'

Young and old doused sticks with kerosene, lit them, and lined up on the grass strip. The pilot landed safely, and everyone helped to unload his precious cargo.

Half an hour later, the first outraged baby squawked as she got her jab of vaccine.

How well does vaccination protect today's Third World children against infectious diseases?

The greatest killers of children in developing countries are diarrhoeal disease and acute respiratory (chest) infection, for many of which we lack good vaccines.

Each year, six preventable diseases (tuberculosis, measles, tetanus, whooping cough, diphtheria, and polio) kill 1.5 million to 2 million children. The measles death rates are about 400 times those of the West.

Almost half a million newborn babies in developing countries die each year of tetanus, an infection that doctors in the West hardly ever see in newborn babies.

This form of tetanus follows lack of immunisation of mothers and contamination during childbirth. Local midwives often cut the umbilical cord with a dirty razor blade, a sliver of bamboo or even a blade of tough grass, and then cover the stump with dung or mud.

The tragedies extend beyond the deaths: each year, there are about 100,000 new victims of polio. Malnutrition, measles, and whooping cough disable many others.

The good news is that each year, increased immunisation is saving the lives of about 3 million children. Childhood measles deaths have fallen from 2 million in 1985 to 1.1 million in 1996.

Since it started in 1974, the Expanded Program on Immunisation (EPI) of the World Health Organisation (WHO) and the United Nations Children's Fund (UNICEF) has been very effective.

For the six diseases mentioned (tuberculosis, measles, tetanus, whooping cough, diphtheria, and polio), EPI has raised the immunisation rate of children under one year of age from 5 per cent to about 80 per cent. This 80 per cent represents over 100 million children.

How can underdeveloped countries around the globe get imported heat-sensitive vaccines to children in isolated villages, and keep the vaccines potent?

To keep up the vital 'cold chain', some countries use solar-powered refrigerators, but most rely on insulated boxes of ice or carbon dioxide. Heat-sensitive markers turn blue if the temperature rises above 10 degrees Celsius.

During the civil war in El Salvador, guerilla leaders agreed to a cease-fire; for 'three days of tranquillity', the only shots fired were of vaccines. When Turkey organised a national immunisation day, civil servants, including the military, helped to immunise children.

Is it worthwhile? Is it cost-effective? Can the world afford such intricate chains to continue the necessary mass campaigns?

To give one child one extra year of life by measles immunisation costs 40 cents; one extra year of life in the USA by treating high blood pressure costs $10,000.

Critics of immunisation and other public-health measures claim that saving the lives of young Third World children is futile if they simply die of other causes soon after. UNICEF accepts the need for other measures as well. To improve child health, UNICEF works towards seven priorities, the acronym of which is GOBIFFF:

- Growth monitoring (weight and height)
- Oral rehydration for diarrhoeal disease
- Breast feeding
- Immunisation
- Food
- Female literacy
- Family planning

Every Third World problem interacts with the others: drought, floods, war, defence spending, poverty, corrupt governments, malnutrition, disposal of sewage and industrial waste, polluted drinking water, illiteracy, high death rates of mothers and children, high birth rates, overpopulation, and environmental damage.

One link is crucial: that between child deaths, birth rate and population growth in developing countries.

It may seem natural to believe that improvement in health care is futile, because it only causes a fall in death rates, and therefore a population explosion. This belief *sounds* plausible, and can too easily become a justification for us in the West to deny aid to the Third World.

But there is strong evidence to the contrary: as they become confident that most of their children will survive, parents gradually have fewer children.

As UNICEF says, there is no conflict between meeting the needs of people and controlling the growth of population.

In 1960, many developing countries had high mortality rates for children under five years (between 200 and 350 deaths per 1000 live births). When these death rates first started to fall, birth rates did not all respond at once. But once child mortality fell below about 150, births also fell.

By now, most Asian and Latin American countries have passed through this initial phase: they are approaching or entering the stage when further falls in child deaths will bring much steeper falls in births.

Maurice Strong, Secretary of the 1992 World Conference on Environment and Health in Rio de Janeiro, summed up: 'The effort to reduce child illness and malnutrition ... is crucial, not only for its own sake, but ... to slow population growth and make possible sustainable development in the 21st century and beyond.'

Critics point out that the world population is still rising, and that falling mortality may be associated with (but not the cause of) falling birthrates. Even so, there is convincing evidence that aid and better health care need not cause a population explosion.

The case for wider use of family planning appears overwhelming. Each year, half a million women die from causes related to pregnancy and childbirth. There is also a ripple effect: many infants in developing countries do not survive the early death of their mother.

Four types of pregnancy are especially dangerous for both mother and child: too young, too old, too many, or too close. That is, when the mother is under 18 or over 35 years old, and has already had four children or has had her last child within two years.

UNICEF estimates that if all births could be spaced at least two years apart, this single change would reduce maternal deaths by about 30 per cent, and child deaths by 20 per cent.

The potential for greater use of family planning is enormous.

One simple contraceptive method is full breast-feeding for four to six months, which also protects infants from many infectious diseases.

But there are many obstacles to the spread of effective contraception. For example, to promote their infant formulas, multinational companies are exploiting the fear of AIDS being transmitted by breast-feeding.

Reportedly it was pressure from the Vatican that removed birth control from the agenda at the Earth Summit in Rio.

Just as problems of children in the Third World are varied, but closely linked, so must be our efforts to relieve them. Priorities should include immunisation, family planning, female literacy, raising the status of women, and the relief of poverty.

(GB)

Bibliography

Chapter 1: Kings and Queens

Bernier, O., *The Secrets of Marie Antoinette*, Fromm, New York, 1985.

Bindoff, S.T., *Tudor England*, Viking (Penguin), Harmondsworth, 1951.

Brewer, C., *The Medical History of the Kings and Queens of England*, self published, London, 1996.

Clarke, John, *The Life and Times of George III*, Weidenfeld & Nicolson, London, 1972.

Dale, Marshall, *Medical Biographies: The Ailments of Thirty-Three Famous Persons*, University of Oklahoma Press, Norman and London, 1987.

Dean, Geoffrey, letter to *British Medical Journal*, 1968, vol. 2, pp. 243–44.

Ellis, H., 'Royal operations', *Medico Legal Journal*, 1969, vol. 37, pp. 97–109.

Erickson, C., *To The Scaffold: The Life of Marie Antoinette*, William Morrow & Co., New York, 1991.

Hurst, Lindsay, 'Porphyria revisited', *Medical History*, 1982, issue 26, pp. 179–82.

Larousse Encyclopedia of Modern History, Larousse, Paris, 1964.

Macalpine, Ida & Hunter, Richard, 'Porphyria in the royal houses of Stuart, Hanover, and Prussia: a follow-up study of George III's illness', *British Medical Journal*, 6 January 1968, vol. 1, pp. 7–18.

Macalpine, Ida & Hunter, Richard, 'The "insanity" of King George III: a classic case of porphyria', *British Medical Journal*, 1966, vol. 1, pp. 65–71.

Macalpine, Ida & Hunter, Richard, *George III and the Mad-Business*, Allen Lane (Penguin), London, 1969.

Medvei, V.C., 'The illness and death of Mary Tudor', *Journal of Royal Society of Medicine*, 1987, vol. 80, p. 766.

Plumb, J.H., Foreword, in Geoffrey Parker, *Philip II*, Hutchinson, London, 1978.

Plumb, J.H., *The First Four Georges*, Little, Brown & Go, Boston, 1975.

Sobrino, L.G., et al., 'Hyperprolactinaemia in women with paternal deprivation in childhood', *Obstet Gynaecology*, 1984, vol. 64, p. 465.

van Loon, Hendrik, *Van Loon's Lives*, Simon & Schuster, New York, 1942.

Chapter 2: Eccentrics, Reformers and Pioneers

Briant, K., *Marie Stopes, A Biography*, Hogarth Press, London, 1962.

Burt, Cyril, *The Gifted Child*, Hodder & Stoughton, London, 1975.

Cohn, Victor, *Sister Kenny, the Woman who Challenged the Doctors*, University of Minnesota Press, Minneapolis, 1975.

Gillie, A., 'Elizabeth Blackwell and the medical register from 1858', *British Medical Journal*, 1958, vol. ii, pp. 1253–57.

Grace, P., 'First among women', *British Medical Journal*, 1991, vol. 303, pp. 1582–83.

Hall, R., *Marie Stopes, A Biography*, Andre Deutsch, London, 1977.

Kevles, Daniel J., *In the Name of Eugenics: Genetics and the Uses of Human Heredity*, Knopf, New York, 1985.

Manton, J., *Elizabeth Garrett Anderson*, Methuen & Go, London, 1965.

Morgan, E.S., *A Short History of Medical Women in Australia*, Burroughs Wellcome, Sydney, 1970.

Rae, Isobel, *The Strange Story of Dr James Barry, Army Surgeon, inspector-General of Hospitals, Discovered on Death to be a Woman*, Longmans Green, London, 1958.

Stopes, M.C., *Married Love*, A.C. Fifield, London, 1918.

Wainer, Bertram, *It Isn't Nice*, Alpha Books, Sydney, 1972.

White, Paul, *Alias Jungle Doctor: An Autobiography*, Paternoster Press, Exeter, 1977.

Chapter 3: Quacks, Pseudologists and Other Phonies

Haggard, H.W., *Devils, Drugs and Doctors*, Blue Ribbon Books, New York, 1929.

Newman, Art, *The Illustrated History of Medical Curiosa*, McGraw-Hill, New York, 1988.

Porter, D. & Porter, R., *Patient's Progress*, Polity Press, London, 1989.

Chapter 4: Famous Patients

Bennett, A., *Writing Home*, Faber & Faber, London, 1994.

Cecil, D., *A Portrait of Jane Austen*, Constable, London, 1978.

Cope, Z., 'Jane Austen's last illness', *British Medical Journal*, 1964, vol. 5402, pp. 182–83.

Crome, L., 'The medical history of V.I. Lenin', *History of Medicine*, 1972, vol. 4, no. 2, pp. 20–22.

Ellmann, R., *Oscar Wilde*, Hamish Hamilton, London, 1987.

Gordon, Richard, *The Great Medical Mysteries of History*, Arrow, 1985.

Halprin, J., *The Life of Jane Austen*, Harvester Press, Brighton, 1984.

Hedayati., H, Barmada, R. & Skosey, J., 'Acrolysis in pachydermoperiostosis', *Archives of Internal Medicine*, 1980, vol. 140, PP. 1087–88.

Khrushchev, N.S., *Khrushchev Remembers*, Andre Deutsch, London, 1971.

Major, R.H., *Classic Description of Disease*, Blackwell, Oxford, 1948.

Moran, Charles (Lord Moran), *Winston Churchill: The Struggle for Survival*, Constable, London; 1966.

Noguchi, Thomas, *Coroner at Large*, Simon & Schuster, New York, 1985.

Payne, R., *The Rise and Fall of Stalin*, Avon Books, New York, 1965.

Sykes, Adam & Sproat, Ian, *The Wit of Sir Winston*, Leslie Frewin, London, 1965.

Taylor, B., 'J. Stalin: a medical case history', *MD State Medical Journal*, November 1975, PP. 35–46.

Thomas, Hugh, *Hess: A Tale of Two Murders*, Hodder & Stoughton, London, 1988.

van Loon, Hendrik, *Van Loon's Lives*, Simon & Schuster, New York, 1942.

Chapter 5: Warfare and Medicine

Crumplin, M.K., 'Surgery at Waterloo', *Journal of the Royal Society of Medicine*, January 1988, 81(1), pp. 38–42.

Dalton, C., *The Waterloo Roll Call*, Arms and Armour Press, London, 1971.

Huxley, Elspeth, *Florence Nightingale*, Weidenfeld & Nicholson, London, 1975.

Richardson, R.G., *Larrey: Surgeon to Napoleon's Imperial Guard*, John Murray, London, 1974.

Chapter 6: Discoveries and Diseases

Bernstein, B.J., 'The swine fever immunization program', *Medical Heritage*, 1985, vol. 1, no. 236–66.

Cleland, J. & Southcott, R.V., Hypervitaminosis A in the Antarctica in the Australian Antarctic Expedition of 1911–1914: a possible explanation of the illnesses of Mertz and Mawson, *The Medical Journal of Australia*, 1969, vol. 1, no. 26, pp. 1337–42.

Eron, C., *The Virus that Ate Cannibals*, Macmillan, New York, 1981, pp. 105–36.

Fraser, Antonia (ed.), *The Lives of the Kings and Queens of England*, Futura, London, 1977.

Howell, Michael & Ford, Peter, *Medical Mysteries*, Viking, London, 1985.

Lindenbaum, S., 'Kuru sorcery', in R.W. Hornabrook (ed.), *Essays on Kuru*, E.W. Classey, Faringdon, Berks, 1976, pp. 28–37.

Woodforde, John, *The Strange Story of False Teeth*, Routledge & Kegan Paul, London, 1968.

Chapter 7: Disasters

Caulfield, Catherine, *Multiple Exposures: Chronicles of the Radiation Age*, Secker & Warburg, London, 1989.

Gordon, R., *Great Medical Disasters*, Hutchinson, London, 1983. Hills, Ben, *Blue Murder, Two Thousand Doomed to Die: The Shocking Truth About Wittenoom's Deadly Dust*, Sun Books, Melbourne, 1989.

Jones, James H., *Bad Blood: The Tuskegee Syphilis Experiment*, The Free Press, New York, 1993.

Nikiforuk, Andrew, *The Fourth Horseman: A Short Account of Epidemics, Plagues and Other Scourges*, Fourth Estate, London, 1991.

O'Brien, Màire & O'Brien, Conor Cruise, *Ireland: A Concise History* (3rd revd edn), Thames & Hudson, New York, 1985.

Schapiro, J. Salwyn, *Modern and Contemporary European History*, Houghton Mifflin, Cambridge, Mass., 1953.

Woodham-Smith, Cecil, *The Great Hunger, Ireland 1845–49*, Hamish Hamilton, London, 1962.

Chapter 8: Addictions and Obsessions

Bird, J., *Percy Grainger*, Elek Books, London, 1976.

Freud, Sigmund, *The Cocaine Papers*, Robert Byck (ed.), New American Library, New York, 1974.

O'Shea, J.G., 'Percy Grainger', *Medical Journal of Australia*, 1987, vol. 1578–1581.

Ober, W.B., *Boswell's Clap and Other Essays: A Medical Analysis of Literary Men's Afflictions*, Southern Illinois University Press, Carbondale, 1979.

Shannon, R., *Gladstone*, vol. I: 1809–1865, Hamish Hamilton, London, 1982.

Waldorf, Dan, *Cocaine Changes: The Experience of Using and Quitting*, Temple University Press, Philadelphia, 1991.

Chapter 9: Longevity

Brewer's Dictionary of Phrase and Fable, E.H. Evans (ed.), Cassell, London, 1981.

Copeman, Herbert, 'Henry Leighton Jones and his contribution to gland grafting', *Medical Journal of Australia*, 1977, vol. 2, pp. 868–71.

Fraser, A., *King Charles II*, Weidenfield & Nicolson, London, 1979.

Kurtzman, J. & Gordon, P., *No More Dying*, Dell, New York, 1977.

Leaf, A., *Youth in Old Age*, McGraw-Hill, New York, 1975.

Stout, R., *et al.*, 'Better ageing: longer useful life', *Update*, 1993, vol. 47, no. 9, pp. 583–595.

Sydney Morning Herald, 15 November 1997.

Weekly Telegraph, issue 138, February 1994.

Young, Harvey James, *The Medical Messiahs*, Princeton University Press, Princeton, New Jersey, 1967.

A Final Word

Goodfield, Jane, *The Planned Miracle*, Scribners, London, 1991.